THE COMPLETE

SLIMMER CLUBS

GUIDE

THE COMPLETE
SLIMMER CLUBS
GUIDE

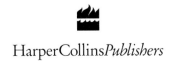

HarperCollins*Publishers*

First published in 1995 by
HarperCollins*Publishers*
77-85 Fulham Palace Road
London W6 8JB

© SP Creative Design 1995

A CIP catalogue for this book is available from the British Library

ISBN 0 00 412745 5

Created and produced by
SP Creative Design
147 Kings Road
Bury St Edmunds
Suffolk IP33 3DJ

Editor: Heather Thomas
Art Director: Al Rockall
Designer: Rolando Ugolini
Slimmer Clubs UK Marketing Manager: Margaret Turner
Slimmer Clubs UK Diet and Nutrition Manager: Tanya May

Photographs
Edward Allright: pages 47, 57, 60, 70
Henry Arden: back cover and page 135
Steve Baxter: pages 44, 45, 114, 115, 116, 117, 118, 119, 120, 121, 122, 123, 124, 125, 126, 127, 130
Gareth Boden: pages 21, 105
Fresh Fruit and Vegetable Information Bureau: page 15
GGS Photographics (Des Adams): pages 12, 13, 18, 19, 34, 35, 38, 42, 50, 53, 54, 55, 58, 64, 65, 69, 73, 74, 75, 94, 95, 100, 101, 106, 107, 110, 111, 128, 129
Colin Gotts: page 134
Graham Kirk: page 91
Steve Lee: pages 48, 87, 88
Polygram Video: back cover and page 113

Acknowledgements
The publishers would like to thank Diana Moran for devising the exercise programme and appearing in the work-out photographs in this book.
Also Reebok UK Ltd for supplying the shoes used in the exercise section and Skinflex (UK) Ltd for supplying the leotards and exercise-wear. Our thanks also to Melanie Faldo PR and Marketing for arranging the exercise photography.

Printed and bound in Italy by New Interlitho Italia SpA, Milan

Contents

FOREWORD

by Tony and Chris Jones, Managing Directors Slimmer Clubs UK

Last year alone, 55,000 people lost more than 700,000 pounds of excess weight while following our diet. Within this book, you will find a diet that's right for you – a diet that will help you lose those unwanted pounds for ever.

As former overweight people ourselves, we know only too well how it feels to make excuses when you have a weight problem. You may find it reassuring to know that we too have refused to remove our jackets when the weather was hot, have lied about our weight and refused social invitations because of our size.

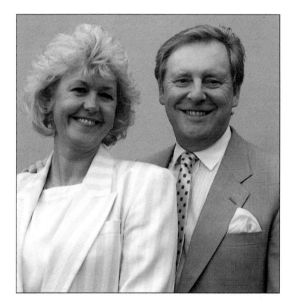

In the past, we have tried all sorts of dieting methods from pills and potions to strenuous jogging, but all to no avail. It was only when we both decided to lose weight sensibly while following a low-fat, low-calorie diet that we understood that dieting really could be fun and, more importantly, that we could maintain that weight loss long-term. With our diet, you too will find that you don't have to go without the foods that you love, because with our 'no forbidden foods' policy you will be able to enjoy the good things in life such as chocolate and wine – and still lose weight!

For the first time, in this book, we are sharing the secrets of our diet so that our success today can be your success tomorrow. Hundreds of thousands of people have lost weight in our weekly classes and have discovered the joys of being fitter, healthier and happier. And, remember, you are not alone. If you need help, then you can always join one of our classes or telephone our Hotline (see page 143).

As you embark upon this challenge to lose weight, take this book in both hands, read the inspirational stories of our successful slimmers and start your diet now! They say that 'life begins at forty' – we feel that life begins when you reach your target weight!

We did it and so can you. Like us, you'll soon discover that this really could be... **your last diet ever!**

by Dr Michael Spira M.B.B.S., M.R.C.S., L.R.C.P.

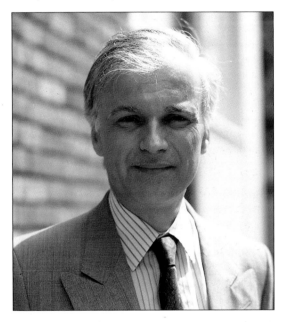

Today there is more confusion about slimming than ever before, and this is at a time when half of all adults are overweight. Why is this?

Slimming requires determination, persistence and, above all, a strong reason why you want to lose weight. Without these, it is difficult to continue with a process that is life-long. The slimming industry has attracted many short-cuts in the form of pills, slimming aids, gadgets and crash diets. These have raised false expectations which are inevitably dashed. Quite rightly, such 'quick fixes' have received much critical media attention, but if a particular slimming method is bad, does this mean that there is no need to slim? Is slimming bad for you?

Of course not. If you are overweight – and this book shows you how to decide this for yourself – you run definite risks to your health. These include high blood pressure, heart disease and stroke, diabetes, arthritis and accidents. The more overweight you are, the greater the risk.

What about the risk of slimming? Providing you have a clear reason why you want to lose weight and you follow a healthy, balanced diet which results in slow but steady weight loss, there is no risk.

Which is why I welcome this book. Here you will find many good reasons for shedding those surplus pounds, and they will provide some ideas for your 'why'. As to the 'how', I know of no more sensible, yet simple, approach to losing weight, which at the same time encourages you to enjoy your food.

A confused mind usually says 'No'. This book takes the confusion out of slimming. As you read it, you will find yourself saying, 'Yes, now I know why I should lose weight. And, yes, now I know how to lose weight.'

Dr Michael Spira is the Medical Consultant to Slimmer Clubs UK.

THE LAST DIET YOU'LL EVER NEED

Are you always on a diet? No matter how hard you try to lose weight, you never seem to keep it off and it creeps back on again when you revert back to your normal eating habits. If you can identify with this phenomenon, don't worry, because you're not alone. There are many other people on the dieting merry-go-round, too. This sort of dieting is both frustrating and disheartening, but slimming need not be like this. You can lose weight and stay slim – permanently!

At Slimmer Clubs UK, our range of simple no-nonsense diets are:

■ Balanced nutritionally and in line with Government health findings.

■ Medically approved and safe for you to follow.

■ Infinitely flexible so that you can continue eating your favourite foods, albeit in moderation.

■ Low in fat and calorie controlled to encourage long-term successful weight loss

■ Filling so that you need never feel hungry or deprived.

■ Individually calorie-counted to cater for the amount of weight you have to lose.

Change your diet now

All our calorie-counted diets are:

■ **Simple to follow:** There are no complicated rules or recipes.

■ **Inexpensive:** There is no need to buy 'special' diet foods and products.

■ **Quick and easy:** There is no need to spend long hours in the kitchen preparing meals.

■ **Varied:** You can choose from a wide range of different menu plans, recipes and convenience foods.

■ **Designed to fit into today's busy lifestyle:** You can stay on your diet plan even if you are working and can't prepare 'special' food at lunchtimes.

■ **Suitable for entertaining or eating out:** You don't have to worry about ruining your diet when you have guests or eat out in a restaurant.

■ **Suitable for sharing with all the family:** The recipes are so delicious that they can eat the same dishes as you and there is no need to cook separate meals for yourself.

■ **Substantial and filling:** Because you feel full up, you are better able to stick to the diet and to continue to lose weight.

The feel-good factor

Following our diet plans will not only help you to lose weight; it will make you feel better, too. As you get trimmer and slimmer, you will feel more confident about yourself, and less self-conscious about your body and your looks.

If you have been very overweight, there will be additional benefits. For example, you will feel less breathless and lethargic, and your joints will move more easily. Many women report that their skin improves – it looks clearer and more radiant – and their hair is more glossy.

For some people, losing weight literally gives them a new lease of life. Our successful slimmers are living testimony to the fact that losing weight can transform your whole life – for the better.

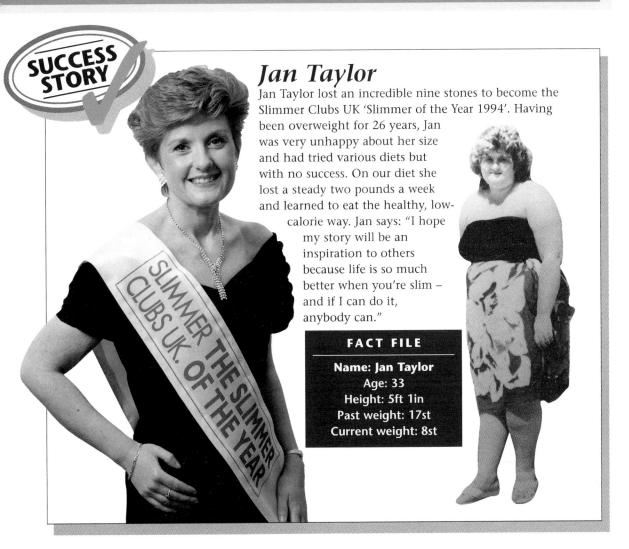

SUCCESS STORY

Jan Taylor

Jan Taylor lost an incredible nine stones to become the Slimmer Clubs UK 'Slimmer of the Year 1994'. Having been overweight for 26 years, Jan was very unhappy about her size and had tried various diets but with no success. On our diet she lost a steady two pounds a week and learned to eat the healthy, low-calorie way. Jan says: "I hope my story will be an inspiration to others because life is so much better when you're slim – and if I can do it, anybody can."

FACT FILE

Name: Jan Taylor
Age: 33
Height: 5ft 1in
Past weight: 17st
Current weight: 8st

Exercise your options

While our diets will help you to lose weight and become more healthy, regular exercise will speed up the process. It burns up calories, and trims and firms slack muscles, and those awkward areas such as hips, thighs, bottom and stomach. It is never too late to start exercising even if you have never exercised before, and fitness expert Diana Moran has designed a special exercise programme (page 112) which you can follow at home.

Believe in yourself

To be successful at losing weight, you must believe that you can do it. Before you embark on your diet, make a personal commitment to losing weight and to stay with the diet. It is important to stick to your resolve and to follow the diet through to the end. Don't be tempted to give up after a few days if you are disappointed with your initial weight loss; successful dieting takes time and requires patience and motivation.

With the diets in this book you will find that dieting is enjoyable as well as simple. To inspire you, just look at the Slimmer Clubs UK real-life success stories in this book. *They did it – and so can you!*

THE IDEAL WEIGHT FOR YOU

You have decided that you want to lose weight and embark on one of our Slimmer Clubs diets, but how much weight should you lose? Before you start, you need to set yourself a goal so that you have a positive and tangible target. With this in mind, we have devised a healthy Height/Weight Chart (see opposite). We advise that you aim for the Suggested Weight within the healthy range of minimum and maximum weights for your height.

Your starting weight

This will determine which diet you choose and how many calories you will eat. All our diets are based on daily calorie intake, and in this book you will find detailed diets and menu plans for the following:

- 1050 calories.
- 1200 calories.
- 1350 calories.
- 1500 calories.
- 1650 calories.

As a general rule, the more weight you have to lose, the higher the calorie intake required for steady long-term weight loss. Crash dieting and starving yourself are unhealthy and are not sustainable. People who do this usually put back on all the weight they have lost as soon as they stop dieting. It is best to aim for a more gradual weight loss, as you are less likely to put the pounds back on again.

You will need to weigh yourself before you start your diet, and then on a regular basis – say, once a week. Don't be tempted to weigh yourself every day and to become obsessed about your weight loss – this may lead to disappointment and even giving up if the pounds are not falling off as quickly as you hoped.

There will be times when you lose weight more quickly, and others when you seem to reach a plateau and it just sticks (page 108). Everybody experiences these minor setbacks, and you can overcome them, too.

To record your weight accurately, follow these simple rules for weighing yourself:

- Always wear the same clothes and weigh yourself without shoes.
- Always use the same scales. Different ones vary and may give different readings.
- Weigh yourself at the same time of day – when you wake up is a good time.
- Bear in mind that your weight may fluctuate throughout the month or year, depending on such factors as your menstrual cycle and the climate.

Body Mass Index

Like all height/weight charts, ours is based on body mass index (BMI). This literally means 'weight relative to height'. You can work out your own BMI with this simple equation:

Weight in kilos divided by height in metres squared

The healthy range for an adult is somewhere between 20 and 25. If your BMI is less than 20, you may be considered underweight; if it is more than 25, you are considered overweight. A BMI of over 30 is viewed as obese.

SLIMMER CLUBS UK – HEIGHT/WEIGHT CHART

Men

Height m	ft. in.	Weight Minimum st lb	Suggested st lb	Maximum st lb
	5.00	7.13	8.10	9.02
1.55	5.01	8.02	9.00	9.06
	5.02	8.05	9.04	9.10
1.60	5.03	8.09	9.08	10.00
	5.04	8.13	9.13	10.05
1.65	5.05	9.04	10.04	10.10
	5.06	9.08	10.08	11.01
1.70	5.07	9.12	10.13	11.06
	5.08	10.02	11.04	11.11
1.75	5.09	10.06	11.09	12.02
	5.10	10.11	12.00	12.07
1.80	5.11	11.01	12.04	12.12
	6.00	11.05	12.09	13.03
1.85	6.01	11.09	13.00	13.08
	6.02	11.13	13.05	13.13
1.90	6.03	12.04	13.10	14.04
	6.04	12.08	14.00	14.09
1.95	6.05	12.12	14.05	15.00

Women

Height m	ft. in.	Weight Minimum st lb	Suggested st lb	Maximum st lb
	4.08	6.10	7.04	8.00
1.45	4.09	6.13	7.08	8.04
	4.10	7.02	7.12	8.08
1.50	4.11	7.05	8.01	8.12
	5.00	7.08	8.05	9.02
1.55	5.01	7.11	8.08	9.06
	5.02	8.00	8.12	9.10
1.60	5.03	8.04	9.02	10.00
	5.04	8.08	9.07	10.05
1.65	5.05	8.12	9.12	10.10
	5.06	9.02	10.02	11.01
1.70	5.07	9.06	10.06	11.06
	5.08	9.10	10.11	11.11
1.75	5.09	10.00	11.02	12.02
	5.10	10.04	11.07	12.07
1.80	5.11	10.08	11.11	12.12
	6.00	10.12	12.01	13.03
1.85	6.01	11.02	12.06	13.08

NOTES ON CHARTS

■ The weights given include an allowance for clothing.

■ Weights for children aged 10-18 years and for pregnant or lactating (nursing) women MUST be advised by their doctor.

■ It is inadvisable for children under the age of 10 years to diet. If you are worried about your child's weight, consult your doctor and follow his recommendations.

HEALTHY EATING

Eating a healthy diet will help you to lose weight and stay slim – for life! With our diets, you can choose from a vast array of healthy, nutritious foods, which have been tried and tested to give a good weight loss. You may even include some treat foods, in moderation, but it is important to get the balance right to continue in good health.

Our diets have been devised in line with current health recommendations and provide all the nutrients you need to stay healthy. They are:

■ Low in fat.
■ High in complex carbohydrates and fibre.
■ Low in sodium.
■ Low in sugar.
■ Contain sufficient low-fat protein to meet your needs.

Protein

Whether you are losing weight or trying to maintain your weight, it is important that your diet contains sufficient protein, as it is the only nutrient capable of replacing worn-out tissue. For example, the cells lining your stomach need to be replaced every few days. During spurts of growth, or during pregnancy or when recovering from an accident or surgery, more protein than usual is needed.

The equivalent of about 175g (6oz) lean meat would supply most people's needs on a day-to-day basis, but you don't have to eat any meat at all as many other foods also supply protein.

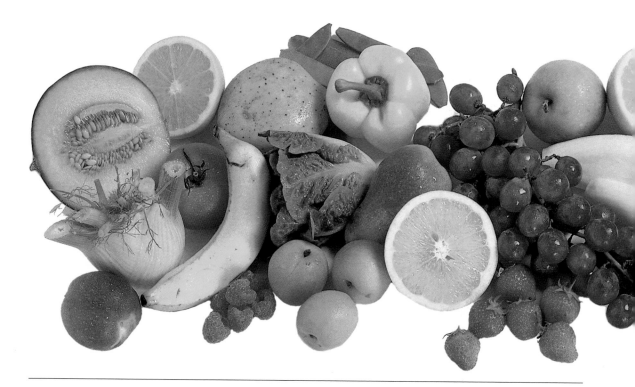

Good sources of protein

Protein is found in both animal and vegetable foods. Poultry, lean meat, fish, skimmed milk, eggs, low-fat cheese and yogurt all provide lots of protein for least calories.

■ Vegetable proteins include whole-grain cereals (e.g. wholemeal bread), grains (e.g. rice), pulses (e.g. beans, peas and lentils), nuts and seeds. To make use of the protein found in vegetable foods, it is necessary to mix different types. For example, beans on toast, chilli beans and rice, chapati and dhal are all traditional mixtures of grains or cereals with pulses. This mixing is needed because most vegetable protein foods lack one of the essential 'amino acids' which are the building blocks of protein. Your body is unable to use any protein unless all the essential amino acids are present in one meal. Mixing them means that there are no missing bits.

Carbohydrates

In the past, carbohydrates were thought to be the slimmer's worst enemy. In part, this was because starches and sugars were all lumped together and also because they were frequently mixed with fat to make high-calorie foods such as cakes and pastry.

■ Starch is found in cereals, grains, and some fruit and vegetables. In their whole form, they are often a good source of vitamins and minerals, and also of fibre which helps to keep everything moving smoothly through our digestive tract. From the slimmer's point of view, they provide a feeling of fullness for a moderate calorie cost.

Along with less starchy fruits and vegetables, they are often referred to as 'complex carbohydrates'. Refined starches, such as white flour, have been stripped of their fibre and much of their vitamin content so provide far less nutrition for the same calories.

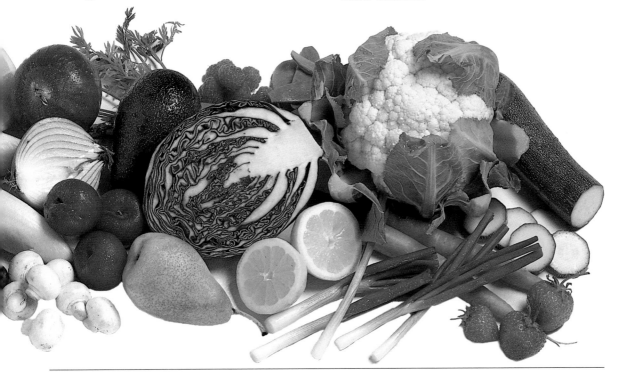

Slimming tip

Try to eat either 450g (1lb) fresh fruit or vegetables a day. This is achieved easily by having a 150g (5oz) piece of fruit, a serving of salad or leafy green vegetables of around 100g (3-4oz) perhaps with your Light Meal, and two servings of other fresh fruit or vegetables, each around 100g (3-4oz) with your Main Meal.

■ Natural sugars are found in many fruits and vegetables, but because of their high water content they are very low in calories. The problems start when natural sugars are processed or refined, and the sugar content gets more concentrated, e.g. dried fruits and fruit juices contain more sugar and calories than whole fruit. Try to avoid foods that contain a lot of added sugar.

Fats

Weight for weight, fats contain more than twice the calories of either protein or carbohydrate. In spite of everything that has been said and written about the effects of too much fat on health, the reality is that most of us still eat too much fat. Even if we have switched to low-fat spreads, milks and cheeses we may still use a lot of fat in cooking or eat foods containing hidden fats, e.g. sausages, pies, nuts, avocados and biscuits.

There are many different types of fat and some are healthier than others. The biggest mistake many people make is to add the healthier fats to their diet without reducing the unhealthy types – so they end up eating even more fat! Saturated fats are the ones to avoid as they tend to be associated with cholesterol problems. These include fatty meats, butter, lard, cream, full-fat cheeses, whole milk and whole-milk yogurt.

We all need just a little polyunsaturated fat to provide the essential fatty acids our bodies can't produce from other fats. It is found mostly in oily fish and vegetable oils.

We all need some fat in our diet in order to absorb and store fat-soluble vitamins, to act as a cushion around vital organs, and to insulate our bodies from the cold. For these reasons, we believe in a low-fat diet, not a no-fat diet!

Vitamins

These are involved in so many different body processes that you could be asking for trouble if you go short on them. Recent research has shown that as well as preventing 'deficiency' diseases, vitamins may play a vital part in protecting us from many so-called affluent diseases associated with heart conditions and certain types of cancer.

There are two types of vitamins: fat-soluble ones which can be stored in the body; and water-soluble ones which need to be replaced daily.

Vitamin A: A fat-soluble vitamin needed for good vision, healthy skin and hair. It can be found in offal, oily fish and eggs. The vegetable form is abundant in yellow and dark green fruits and vegetables such as carrots, fresh or dried apricots, spinach and broccoli.

Vitamin B: This comprises a whole group of water-soluble vitamins, but they are often found together in the same foods. One of their most important functions is to convert food into energy. Good sources are lean pork, offal, whole-grain cereals, brown rice, beans, yeast extract, milk, cheese and eggs.

Cobalamin (B12) is rarely found in vegetable foods so vegans may need a supplement. Folic acid, another B vitamin, is very important during pregnancy and is plentiful in leafy green vegetables as well as the foods already listed.

Vitamin C: This water-soluble vitamin helps our bodies to fight infection and absorb iron. The best sources are citrus fruits (oranges, lemons, grapefruit, tangerines, limes), blackcurrants, strawberries, melon, kiwi fruit, green vegetables, red and green peppers.

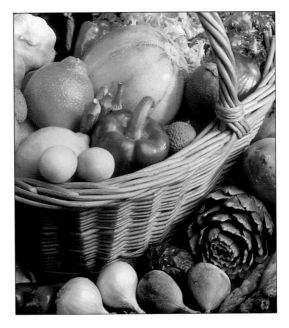

Vitamin D: This fat-soluble vitamin is made by the action of sunlight on our skin. It is found in oily fish, liver, egg yolk and cheese. It is added to margarine and low-fat spreads, and is essential for the absorption of calcium.

Vitamin E: This fat-soluble vitamin helps to maintain healthy red blood cells. It is found in whole grains, vegetable oils and leafy green vegetables.

Vitamin K: A fat-soluble vitamin essential for blood clotting. Cauliflower and leafy green vegetables are good sources.

Vitamin and mineral supplements: If you eat a healthy, balanced diet, you should not need these. In fact, it can be potentially

dangerous to take too many fat-soluble vitamins which are stored in the body. Ask your doctor for advice on this.

Minerals

These are present in many foods and perform a wide range of functions. The most important ones are calcium and iron.

Calcium: This is needed for building strong, healthy bones and teeth, and is especially important in childhood, pregnancy and during the menopause. It is found in milk, cheese, yogurt, the mashed soft bones of oily fish such as sardines, and dark green leafy vegetables. Skimmed milk contains as much calcium as whole milk.

Iron: This is important for making red blood cells. Good sources are offal and lean red meat. Spinach, pulses, whole-grain cereals and dried fruits are good vegetable sources but must be eaten with vitamin C in order to be absorbed.

Slimming tip

A surplus of calories makes you gain weight. A deficit of calories makes you lose weight.

COOKING THE LOW-CALORIE WAY

Eat the low-calorie way

Dieting success can be yours if you eat the healthy, low-calorie way. Use the following tips and guidelines to cut wasted calories and retain maximum nutrients.

Preparing food

■ If you really wish to be successful in losing weight, then weigh and measure out portions of food, at least until you get a good eye for portion size. However, even then you should take care as it is easy to fool yourself. Your 30g (1oz) of cheese could be wildly out and have twice the calories you think you are having. A heaped spoonful can have double the calories of a level spoonful.

■ Trim all visible fat from meat, and skim off any fat which has cooked out of stews and casseroles. Poultry skin is very high in calories but can help to keep white meat moist whilst grilling or roasting – make sure it is removed before eating.

■ Make a little go a long way. By slicing meat really thinly, you can make it appear more. Using frozen meat which is partially defrosted is a good idea as it is easy to cut thinly at this stage. After slicing, continue to defrost completely before cooking.

■ Grate cheese for sandwiches and pizza toppings, or cut wafer-thin slices with a potato peeler. Either way, you will use less cheese than if you try slicing it with a knife.

Cooking food

■ Use natural flavourings. Cut down on the salt you eat; too much is unhealthy and encourages fluid retention. You can substitute herbs and spices, which contain virtually no calories.

■ Retain maximum vitamin content by preparing fruit and vegetables just prior to cooking, and steam, microwave or stir-fry them until just tender but still crisp.

■ Dry-fry mince in its own fat in a non-stick pan, and drain well before adding to a dish.

■ Whenever possible, grill foods. Most meat, oily fish, low-fat burgers or sausages can be grilled in preference to frying. You can save even more calories by draining them on absorbent kitchen paper.

■ Try poaching and cooking en papillote. Fish steaks and fillets and chicken portions are delicious poached in a little stock, or cooked in foil or greaseproof paper with herbs, chopped vegetables and lemon juice.

Eat less fat

If you really want to lose weight and be more healthy, you must cut down on the amount of fat you eat. There are all sorts of special low-fat spreads, yogurts, milk, salad dressings and other products to help you. Here are some general guidelines:

■ Beware of hidden fats. These lurk in many everyday foods, and you may not even be aware of their existence. Common culprits include mayonnaise, salad dressings, crisps, sauces, biscuits, cakes, pastries, chocolate, cheese, nuts and many fast foods, especially take-aways. Eat these foods only occasionally.

■ Opt for lower fat alternatives. Choose skimmed milk, cottage and half-fat cheese, very low-fat fromage frais, low-fat spreads, low-fat diet yogurts and oil-free or reduced-calorie salad dressings in place of regular brands.

■ Use less fat in cooking. Many of your favourite recipes will work just as well if you reduce the fat in them. For example, you can fry vegetables in a teaspoon of oil; you can use half-fat cheese for toppings before baking or grilling; and pastry can be made with low-fat spread.

■ Cut out cream. You do not have to top desserts, fruit and puddings with cream. Low-fat diet yogurts and very low-fat fromage frais make delicious substitutes.

Eat less sugar

Most of us have a sweet tooth, but sugar is 'empty' calories and has little or no nutritional value. If you are to get slim and stay that way, you must cut down on sugar. Here are some tips to help you:

■ Use artificial sweetener in place of sugar in drinks if you really need to. You can also use granulated sweeteners in desserts at the end of cooking. Some lose their sweetness on heating, so check labels before using in a recipe.

What is a calorie?

In dieting terms, a calorie is simply a unit of measurement for the amount of energy in food. Nowadays it is often called a kilocalorie. Don't be confused by kilojoules; they are just the metric version (approximately 4 kilojoules equal 1 kilocalorie).

If you are gaining weight, it is because you are supplying your body with more energy than it can use up and so it is storing it as fat. If you eat fewer calories than your body needs, then it will use up those surplus fat stores and you will lose weight.

There are approximately 3500 calories in 450g (1lb) of fat weight. Each time you accumulate a spare 3500 calories, you will gain a pound of fat. Each time you accumulate a deficit of 3500 calories, you will lose a pound of fat. It is a paradox that the amount of weight you lose depends not on the number of calories you eat, but on the number of calories you don't eat!

■ Opt for low-calorie diet drinks, mineral waters or unsweetened fruit juices rather than sugary drinks.

■ Keep alcohol within recognised health limits. A man should consume no more than 21 units per week; a woman no more than 14 per week. Keep two days a week alcohol-free. A 'unit' is 275ml ($^{1}/_{2}$ pint) beer or cider, a glass of wine, a single pub measure of sherry, spirits or liqueur.

■ Choose reduced-sugar baked beans or spaghetti in tomato sauce.

NEXT-TO-NOTHING FOODS

All the foods featured here are extremely low in calories, and therefore can be eaten as healthy snacks and fillers without worrying about your waistline. Of course, if you add sugar to fruit or oily dressings or mayonnaise to vegetables, you will be adding unwanted calories.

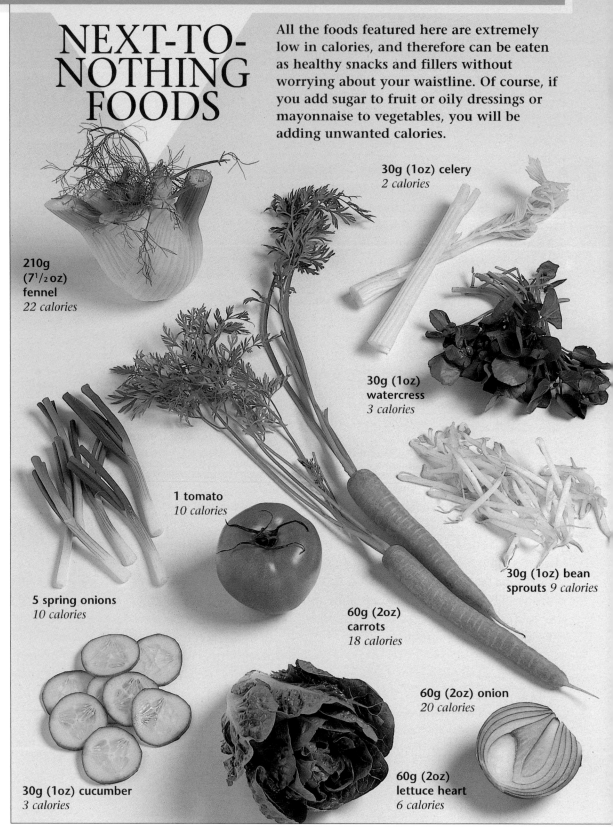

210g (7¹/₂oz) fennel
22 calories

30g (1oz) celery
2 calories

30g (1oz) watercress
3 calories

1 tomato
10 calories

30g (1oz) bean sprouts *9 calories*

5 spring onions
10 calories

60g (2oz) carrots
18 calories

60g (2oz) onion
20 calories

30g (1oz) cucumber
3 calories

60g (2oz) lettuce heart
6 calories

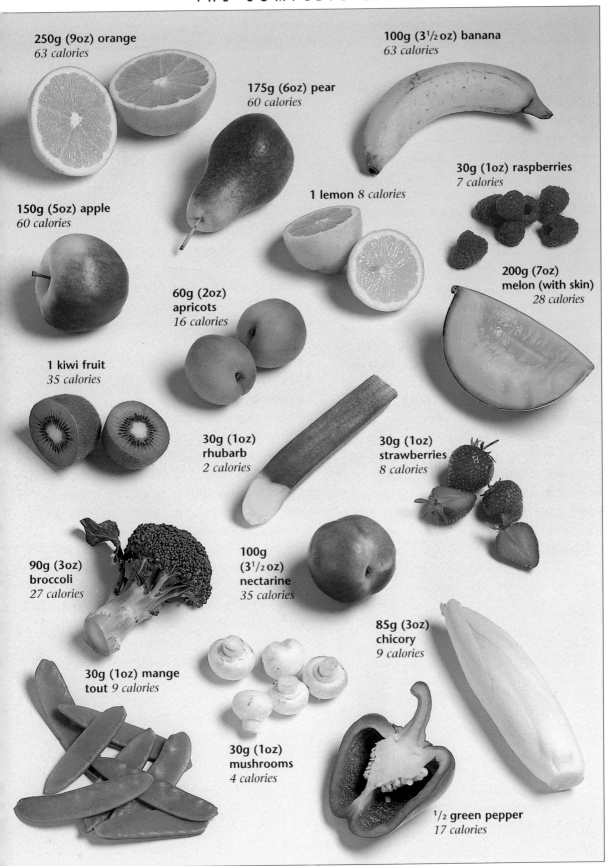

250g (9oz) orange
63 calories

100g (3½oz) banana
63 calories

175g (6oz) pear
60 calories

30g (1oz) raspberries
7 calories

150g (5oz) apple
60 calories

1 lemon *8 calories*

200g (7oz) melon (with skin)
28 calories

60g (2oz) apricots
16 calories

1 kiwi fruit
35 calories

30g (1oz) rhubarb
2 calories

30g (1oz) strawberries
8 calories

90g (3oz) broccoli
27 calories

100g (3½oz) nectarine
35 calories

85g (3oz) chicory
9 calories

30g (1oz) mange tout *9 calories*

30g (1oz) mushrooms
4 calories

½ green pepper
17 calories

Discover vegetables

Vegetables are the greatest ally you have in your personal quest to lose weight and eat a healthier diet. With the exception of potatoes and the starchy vegetables (e.g. parsnips, sweetcorn), most vegetables are very low in calories and rich in vitamins and minerals.

■ **They bulk out meals:** You need never feel hungry if you bulk out your meal with low-calorie vegetables (see the list on page 24). You can eat most vegetables freely and they will add interest and diversity to your diet.

■ **They add dietary fibre and nutrients:** You can maintain their maximum vitamin content by storing them out of the light and not for too long. Only peel and chop them immediately before eating or cooking as some vitamins oxidize quickly on exposure to air. The best way to cook vegetables is to steam them; otherwise add to boiling water and cook until they are tender but still crisp.

■ **Experiment with salads:** There is more to salads than limp lettuce, tomato and soggy cucumber. You can use a wide range of vegetables, fruit and beans, and toss them in a low-calorie dressing. Salads should be crunchy, colourful and delicious, and you will find some unusual recipes in this book. Ring the changes with different ready-made low-calorie dressings, or make your own with the minimum of oil, adding lemon or lime juice, vinegar and herbs. You can also make sumptuous dressings with diet fromage frais and yogurt.

■ **Make satisfying soups:** Vegetable soups are filling and warming in winter, or can be served chilled in summer. They are easy to make and a good low-calorie way to bulk out a meal. They can also be eaten as snacks, using your daily Extras allowance. The Mixed Vegetable Soup recipe on page 76 is particularly good and low in calories. You can make soups in bulk and then freeze them in individual portions until needed.

■ **Use vegetables as snacks:** Don't be tempted to grab a chocolate bar or biscuit when you feel like a snack – eat some raw vegetables instead. Red and green peppers, mushrooms, cauliflower and broccoli florets, carrots and celery sticks, radishes and chunks of cucumber can all be kept in the fridge, and then nibbled as a snack or served as crudités with a low-calorie fromage frais, yogurt or cottage cheese dip.

■ **Be adventurous:** Try out some of the more interesting and exotic-looking vegetables on the shelves of your local supermarket. Have fun cooking with okra, aubergines, cho-cho (christophene), chicory, romanesco cauliflower, purple sprouting broccoli etc. You can also try out the more unusual salad vegetables, such as curly endive (frisée), radicchio and rocket.

Slimming tip

Lots of people, especially children and young people, claim that they don't like any vegetables and never eat them, but there are so many to choose from with such a wide range of shapes, colours, textures and flavours that if they persevere they are bound to discover something they like. Be bold and adventurous and have fun trying out new vegetables. To make them more interesting, try stir-frying them with herbs and spices.

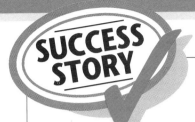

SUCCESS STORY ✓

Ray and Helen Harris

Between them, Ray and Helen Harris have lost an incredible 13 stones in weight. Ray reached his target within 12 months while Helen took 15 months. Before taking the plunge and joining Slimmer Clubs UK, they both ate large cooked breakfasts, at least three roast meals a week, puddings, cakes, and a packet of biscuits per night! They would even eat at home before they went out for a meal. However, they have now learnt to prepare healthy, low-fat meals.

Ray says: "Much to my amazement, I found the healthy foods really enjoyable. No more just stuffing food in and feeling blown-out and exhausted...Although Helen and I were always fat and happy together, it's so great to be slim, happy and healthy instead. Life's getting better and better!"

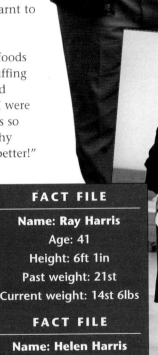

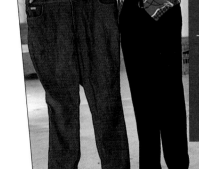

FACT FILE
Name: Ray Harris
Age: 41
Height: 6ft 1in
Past weight: 21st
Current weight: 14st 6lbs

FACT FILE
Name: Helen Harris
Age: 37
Height: 5ft 2in
Past weight: 15st 10lbs
Current weight: 9st 5lbs

CHOOSING YOUR DIET

Now that you have decided that you really want to lose weight, you have to choose the diet that will work best for you. So which diet should you choose? At Slimmer Clubs UK we have devised five different diets, which are all flexible and give you plenty of choice, so that you can continue eating many of your favourite foods.

Generally speaking, a heavier person needs more calories than a lighter person, and therefore can lose weight on a higher calorie intake. Use the chart below as a guide to the level of calories on which you should START dieting.

Most people will lose between two and seven pounds during the first week of their diet. This is partly due to fluid loss. After the euphoria of the first week's successful weight loss subsides, you should expect to lose in the region of one to two pounds a week. Our experience shows that slow and steady weight loss is best and will achieve the best results long-term. Crash diets may provide rapid weight loss in the short-term, but people soon regain the lost pounds when they return to their old eating habits. This form of dieting, more often than not, leads to a vicious cycle of losing and gaining weight so that people are always dieting. The only successful way to lose weight is to eat a healthier diet which is lower in calories, fat and sugar. The diets and information in this book will show you how to do this, so that you can get slim and stay slim – for life!

Which diet?

Look at the chart below and decide which starting level is most appropriate for you. Follow the chosen diet as outlined in the following pages, and stick with it. If you are really following your diet closely but do not seem to be losing weight (between one and two pounds a week is sensible), then try dropping down to the next level.

Important: Women should not drop below 1,000 to 1,050 calories per day; and men

Finding your starting level

Starting weight	Starting daily calories
Women:	
Under 10.00 stones	1050
10.00 – 12.00 stones	1200
12.01 – 14.00 stones	1350
14.01 – 18.00 stones	1500
Over 18.00 stones	1650
Men:	
Under 15.00 stone	1500
Over 15.00 stones	1650

Note: These calorie levels are not appropriate for children under 18 years, nor for women who are pregnant or lactating (nursing mothers). They should consult with, and gain the advice and approval of, their doctor before commencing any weight-loss diet.

Important: If you have any medical condition or are taking medication, you should check with your doctor before commencing any weight-loss diet.

should not drop below 1,200 to 1,350 calories daily. It is very difficult to meet your nutritional needs below these levels. Because your energy requirements tend to adapt to the amount of calories you eat most often, it is self-defeating to eat too little. It will only leave you feeling drained and exhausted.

No forbidden foods

At Slimmer Clubs, we believe very strongly that there is no such thing as a bad food – only a bad diet. In other words, with our diets, no specific foods are expressly forbidden, but, of course, as in all things some moderation is required. Therefore, you are encouraged to eat healthy, nutritious foods most of the time, but you can have 'treat' foods in small amounts occasionally.

A flexible diet plan

For each level of calories, we have set out seven daily menu plans. Within each plan, you will find alternative choices to cater for different food preferences and lifestyles. For example, on at least five of the seven days, you will find a packed lunch alternative if you are at work or college and unable to prepare or cook a light lunch.

There are also alternative menus for vegetarians and people who don't eat red meat. Thus the main meal choices include a quick and easy 'basic' meal for people in a hurry, a vegetarian alternative, and a recipe meal. Once a week, there is a possible 'meal out' choice, just in case you are going out to dinner and need advice on choosing a slimming, healthy dish from the menu in the restaurant, or even ordering in a take-away meal. For more advice on this, see page 96.

If you choose to cook the recipe meal,

there is no need to cook separate food for the rest of the family. Most of the recipes serve four, and are suitable for everyone. For the family members who are not slimming, just add extra bread, rice, pasta or potatoes to their meals.

You can increase your choice further by swapping a meal of equal calorie value from one of the other diets if wished. You may even decide to change the order of your Light and Main Meals, and eat your Main Meal at lunchtime. This is OK as long as you stay within the calorie limits for that day. However, you must not be tempted to skip breakfast. This is a very important meal when you are dieting, and it will help to keep up your energy levels during the morning and prevent over-eating at lunchtime.

Diet guidelines

Like all diets, there are some basic rules and guidelines which you must follow if you want to be successful and achieve your target weight. These 'rules' will enhance your chances of dieting success, and will help you to stay healthy while losing weight. Read them carefully and always follow them. After a while, they will become second nature to you, and will help you establish healthier eating habits and cooking methods for the future, when the time comes to maintain your new weight and slim figure.

■ Eat a wide variety of different types of food. This will add interest to your diet and prevent it being boring. It will also help make it nutritionally better balanced.

■ Choose wholemeal bread and pasta, and whole-grain cereals and rice whenever possible. These foods are all high in fibre and rich in B vitamins, which help to release the energy from food so that you can burn up the calories instead of storing them!

■ Use herbs and small amounts of spices, e.g. pepper, mustard and curry powder, to flavour food. Be sparing with seasonings such as soy sauce, Worcestershire sauce, stock cubes and salt, especially if you have been advised to follow a low-sodium diet.

■ You may have 2-3 tablespoons of thin low-fat gravy with your meals. Look out for gravy powders and granules which are low in fat, and choose these in preference to other brands.

Drinks

You may drink as much water, mineral water, tea and coffee as you wish. Any milk taken in tea or coffee or used on cereal must come from your daily allowance (see right). You may also drink low-calorie squashes and up to 3 cans (approximately 1 litre in total) of fizzy diet drinks per day.

Milk allowance

This is an important source of protein and calcium in your diet. The daily allowance is listed at the beginning of the diet plan for each day. If you cannot tolerate milk for any reason, you may have an extra 30-60g (1-2oz) lean meat or fish, or 100g (3½oz) cooked beans or peas. You must also eat plenty of leafy green vegetables, such as broccoli, spinach, Brussels sprouts and cabbage.

Alternatively, you may substitute 30g (1oz) half-fat cheese or 2 diet yogurts or fromage frais for each 275ml (½ pint) milk.

Reduce your fat intake

■ The term 'diet yogurt' refers to a 125g (4½oz) carton of diet or virtually fat-free yogurt. The term '1 diet fromage frais' refers to a 100g (3 ½oz) carton of diet or virtually

Vegetables

■ Most vegetables are very low in calories. If you feel hungry at mealtimes, you may have more of the following vegetables than the quantities stated in the diet plan. They will not ruin your diet! You can also choose these vegetables if you have 'run out of calories' and feel that you really must eat something.

■ **Very low-calorie vegetables – 5 or less calories per 30g (1oz)**
A 100g (3 ½oz) serving of the following will provide approximately 15 calories: aubergine, celeriac, celery, chicory, courgettes, cucumber, endive, fennel, lettuce, marrow, mushrooms, mustard and cress, green peppers, pumpkin, radishes, tomatoes.

■ **Low-calorie vegetables – 6-10 calories per 30g (1oz)**
A 100g (3 ½oz) serving of the following will provide approximately 25 calories: artichokes, asparagus, bamboo shoots, baby sweetcorn, beans (green), bean sprouts, broccoli, Brussels sprouts, cabbage, calabrese, carrots, cauliflower, chillies, Chinese leaf, cho-cho, kale, kohlrabi, leeks, mange tout, mooli, okra, onions, peppers (red, orange, purple and yellow), spinach, spring greens, squash, swede, turnip and watercress.

Note: The cooking method used is obviously very important. The healthiest ways to cook vegetables are steaming, grilling, boiling and stir-frying. Roasting or frying in fat will add unwanted calories, and should be avoided.

fat-free or 0-1 per cent fat fromage frais.

■ Yogurts and fromage frais that are labelled simply as 'low-fat' usually contain more added sugar and may have twice the calories of diet yogurts and fromage frais. Always check the labels and nutritional information carefully.

■ Including some fat in your diet is essential for good health, but you should aim to cut out surplus fat which is high in calories and very unhealthy. Therefore, you should always trim all visible fat off meat, remove the skin from chicken, and try to have no more than a maximum of 4 eggs per week (6 for vegetarians). Always choose lower-fat products in preference to high-fat foods.

Reduce your sugar intake

■ Cut out sugar in hot drinks, e.g. tea and coffee. If you really do have a sweet tooth, use artificial sweetener instead.

■ Remember that you can cook with some artificial sweeteners and use them in place of sugar in desserts and some cakes.

■ Opt for diet drinks instead of ones that have been sweetened with sugar.

■ Check the labels on packets of fruit juice etc. Many fruit juice 'drinks' have been sweetened with added sugar.

■ Buy fruit that has been canned in water, or natural fruit juice – not in syrup.

Vegetarians

Being vegetarian means different things to different people. If there are any foods that you prefer not to eat, choose an appropriate alternative. In our Diet Plans, we have provided a vegetarian alternative for each meal: Breakfasts, Light Meals and Main Meals.

Weighing and measuring food

■ This may seem like a chore, especially when you are measuring out very small quantities, but it is essential in the initial stages of your diet if you are going to lose weight successfully. For the best results, you must always weigh or measure food, except where a weight is not specified. Spoon measures throughout are standard, level spoonfuls:

> 1 tablespoon = 15ml
> 1 dessertspoon = 10ml
> 1 teaspoon = 5ml
> $^1/_2$ teaspoon = 2.5ml

■ Unless otherwise stated, raw weights are used throughout. For example, 85g (3oz) lean beef = 85g (3oz) weighed raw; but 60g (2oz) roast beef = 60g (2oz) weighed after cooking.

■ All fruit should be weighed with skin and pips or stones. For example, weigh bananas or melons with the skin on.

Extras

Each diet has a calorie allowance for 'extras'. These are 'free choice' calories which you can either add to a meal OR have as between-meal snacks OR you may save all or part of this allowance to put towards a special treat or a meal out.

They may be chosen from the Calorie Lists at the end of the book (page 136) or you can use the nutritional labels on most branded goods to help you decide which foods can be included in your diet.

1050 CALORIES DIET

10 steps to success

1 You should use this diet as your starting point if you are a woman and currently weigh under 10 stones. Do not be tempted to try this diet if you have a lot of weight to lose, in which case you would be better advised to opt for another diet with a higher daily calorie allowance and to aim for more gradual long-term weight loss.

2 You should choose one Breakfast, one Light Meal and one Main Meal each day from the selections that we have given you. Within each choice of meals, there is a vegetarian option, and within the Light Meal selections, there are meals that you can cook at home or ideas for packed lunches that you can take to work with you.

3 You may eat your Breakfast, Light Meal and Main Meal in any order and at any time to suit your particular needs throughout the day.

4 You should not skip meals, especially Breakfast. Make sure that you eat these three meals every day for a balanced diet.

5 Do not forget that every day you must also have your Milk and Fat Allowance as set out on each page. You may use the Milk Allowance throughout the day in drinks and on cereal and in cooking. You may use the Fat Allowance for spreading on bread or crispbreads, or in salad dressings or for cooking.

6 When following this diet, you may have 100 calories per day to spend as you please. You may use them each day OR save them for a higher calorie item.

7 We have given you a complete week of meal ideas but the diet plan is flexible. You may choose one Breakfast, Light Meal or Main Meal from any of the seven daily plans for this calorie level. You may also substitute a meal from the recipe section (see page 76) for any meal with a similar calorie count.

8 You can drop down to this calorie level of 1050 calories per day if you have previously been consuming 1200 calories per day, or at a time when your motivation is high and you really want to lose weight fast.

9 On the following pages, we have given you suggestions for the food that you need to eat to lose weight, but there is more to losing weight than just eating! If you are just starting to follow this diet, why not also start doing the work-out exercises (see page 112) or take up some other form of exercise?

10 As you start to follow this calorie level, make a note of your weight at the start of the week. It is better if you do not weigh yourself again until the same time next week so that you can see the results of your efforts.

DAY 1

150 CALORIES — MILK AND FAT ALLOWANCE

275ml (¹/₂ pint) skimmed milk
3 teaspoons low-fat spread or 1 teaspoon oil

— OR —

275ml (¹/₂ pint) semi-skimmed milk
2 teaspoons very low-fat spread
or ¹/₂ teaspoon oil

150 CALORIES — BREAKFASTS

30g (1oz) non-sugar-coated cereal plus
150g (5oz) fresh fruit or 85g (3oz) banana or
100g (3¹/₂oz) fruit canned in natural juice or
115ml (4 fl oz) unsweetened citrus juice

250 CALORIES — LIGHT MEALS

Sandwich made from 2 x 20g (³/₄oz)
slices bread
30g (1oz) half-fat cheese
Salad garnish
1 diet yogurt

— OR —

60g (2oz) lean ham
Green salad and tomatoes
150g (5oz) banana
1 diet yogurt or 1 diet fromage frais

400 CALORIES — MAIN MEALS

85g (3oz) skinless chicken breast,
grilled or oven-baked
175g (6oz) new potatoes
100g (3¹/₂oz) Brussels sprouts
100g (3¹/₂oz) carrots
1 peach or pear

— OR —

100g (3¹/₂oz) firm tofu, cubed and sprinkled
with a little soy sauce, then grilled until starting
to brown
60g (2oz) brown rice (raw weight), boiled
100g (3¹/₂oz) frozen mixed vegetables
3 tablespoons passata (sieved tomatoes)
1 peach or pear

— OR —

Tandoori Chicken (see recipe below)
Green salad
45g (1¹/₂oz) rice (raw weight), boiled
1 peach or pear

100 CALORIES — EXTRAS

Anything up to 100 calories. All or part of this
allowance may be saved for another day.

TANDOORI CHICKEN

Ingredients
8 chicken drumsticks, skinned
275ml (¹/₂ pint) low-fat natural yogurt
2 garlic cloves, crushed
2 teaspoons tandoori masala spices
¹/₂ teaspoon chilli powder
1 tablespoon ground coriander
1 teaspoon ground cumin
1 teaspoon salt
2 tablespoons finely chopped coriander

1 Slash the drumsticks diagonally 3 or 4 times with a sharp knife. Stir all the remaining ingredients together in a large bowl, and add the drumsticks. Leave to marinate for 2 hours.

2 Transfer the chicken and marinade mixture to a roasting pan, and cook in a preheated oven at 200°C/400°F/Gas Mark 6 for 20 minutes, until the chicken is cooked and tender. If wished, place the chicken under a hot grill for 2-3 minutes to brown.

Serves 4   *180 calories per serving (2 drumsticks)*

150 CALORIES — MILK AND FAT ALLOWANCE

275ml (¹/₂ pint) skimmed milk
3 teaspoons low-fat spread or 1 teaspoon oil

— OR —

275ml (¹/₂ pint) semi-skimmed milk
2 teaspoons very low-fat spread
or ¹/₂ teaspoon oil

150 CALORIES — BREAKFASTS

¹/₂ grapefruit
2 x 20g (³/₄oz) slices toast
Grilled tomatoes or poached
or microwaved mushrooms

250 CALORIES — LIGHT MEALS

115g (4oz) cottage cheese, natural or with
pineapple, or 1 skinless chicken thigh
Green salad and tomatoes
50g (1³/₄oz) wholemeal roll

— OR —

85g (3oz) pilchards in tomato sauce on
2 x 20g (³/₄oz) slices toast
1 orange

400 CALORIES — MAIN MEALS

Any ready meal or vegetarian ready meal
up to 300 calories
200g (7oz) vegetables from low-calorie list
1 diet yogurt or 1 diet fromage frais

— OR —

Spanish Rice (see recipe page 52)
1 kiwi fruit

100 CALORIES — EXTRAS

Anything up to 100 calories. All or part of this
allowance may be saved for another day.

Spanish Rice

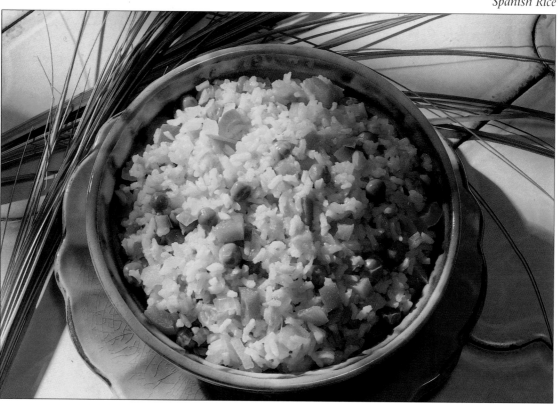

DAY 3

150 CALORIES — MILK AND FAT ALLOWANCE

275ml ($^1/_2$ pint) skimmed milk
3 teaspoons low-fat spread or 1 teaspoon oil

— OR —

275ml ($^1/_2$ pint) semi-skimmed milk
2 teaspoons very low-fat spread
or $^1/_2$ teaspoon oil

150 CALORIES — BREAKFASTS

$^1/_2$ grapefruit
1 size 4 egg, poached or boiled
20g ($^3/_4$oz) slice bread or toast

250 CALORIES — LIGHT MEALS

45g (1$^1/_2$oz) low-fat pâté or vegetarian pâté
3 crispbreads
2 tomatoes
1 orange

— OR —

Any low-calorie soup up to 70 calories
2 x 20g ($^3/_4$oz) slices bread
1 diet fromage frais
1 kiwi fruit

400 CALORIES — MAIN MEALS

85g (3oz) lean trimmed boneless pork chop or
gammon steak, grilled
1 pineapple ring, grilled
85g (3oz) peas
Grilled tomatoes
175g (6oz) potato, jacket baked or microwaved
1 diet yogurt or 150g (5oz) fresh fruit

— OR —

1 Vegeburger, grilled (see recipe page 39)
75g (2$^1/_2$oz) peas
75g (2$^1/_2$oz) cauliflower
175g (6oz) potato, jacket baked or microwaved
1 diet yogurt

— OR —

1 low-calorie Beefburger (see recipe below)
75g (2$^1/_2$oz) peas
Grilled tomatoes
150g (5oz) potato, jacket baked or microwaved
1 diet yogurt or 150g (5oz) fresh fruit

100 CALORIES — EXTRAS

Anything up to 100 calories. All or part of this
allowance may be saved for another day.

LOW-CALORIE BEEFBURGERS

Ingredients
2 slices wholemeal bread, crusts removed and soaked in water
450g (1lb) extra-lean minced beef
1 small onion, grated
3 tablespoons chopped herbs, e.g. parsley, chives, thyme, marjoram
1 garlic clove, crushed
2 teaspoons Worcestershire sauce (optional)
1 teaspoon Dijon mustard
1 egg (size 4), beaten
freshly ground black pepper

1 Squeeze out any excess water from the bread and add to the minced beef with the onion, herbs, garlic, Worcestershire sauce (optional), mustard and beaten egg. Mix well together and season with pepper.

2 Divide the mixture into 4 portions and shape into burgers. Place under a preheated hot grill or on a barbecue until cooked, turning half-way through.

Serves 4 *250 calories per serving*

150 CALORIES — MILK AND FAT ALLOWANCE

275ml (¹/₂ pint) skimmed milk
3 teaspoons low-fat spread or 1 teaspoon oil

OR

275ml (¹/₂ pint) semi-skimmed milk
2 teaspoons very low-fat spread
or ¹/₂ teaspoon oil

150 CALORIES — BREAKFASTS

2 Weetabix or Shredded Wheat or
45g (1¹/₂oz) no-added-sugar muesli

250 CALORIES — LIGHT MEALS

Sandwich made from
2 x 20g (³/₄oz) slices bread
45g (1¹/₂oz) lean corned beef and sliced tomato
or 1 size 4 hard-boiled egg, 1 tablespoon
reduced-calorie salad cream, mustard and cress
1 orange

OR

2 small low-fat sausages, grilled
150g (5oz) reduced-sugar and salt baked beans
1 orange

400 CALORIES — MAIN MEALS

60g (2oz) extra-lean minced beef, dry fried or
microwaved and mixed with 100g (3¹/₂oz)
ready-made pasta sauce
60g (2oz) spaghetti or pasta shapes, boiled
1 teaspoon grated Parmesan cheese
Green side salad

OR

Pasta with Tomato Sauce (see recipe page 86)
1 diet yogurt or 1 diet fromage frais

100 CALORIES — EXTRAS

Anything up to 100 calories. All or part of this
allowance may be saved for another day.

Slimming tip: Pasta

Contrary to popular belief, it is not the pasta that is fattening but the sauce in which it is often served. Pasta is a nutritious food and contains only 40 calories per 30g (1oz) when boiled. However, if it is tossed in a creamy or oily sauce and then sprinkled liberally with Parmesan cheese, the calories will escalate. The recipes in this book will give you some ideas for low-calorie sauces, many of which are tomato and vegetable-based.

Types of pasta

Pasta may be bought dried or fresh. It comes in a seemingly endless array of shapes, sizes and even colours. For example, it can be coloured green with spinach, pink with tomato purée, or even black with cuttlefish ink. It can also be flavoured with the addition of garlic or fresh chopped herbs to the pasta dough.

Cooking pasta

To cook perfect pasta, bring a large saucepan of lightly salted water to a rolling boil and then tip in the pasta and cook until it is *al dente* (tender 'to the bite' but still firm). For fresh pasta, this may take as little as 2-4 minutes; for dry pasta anything from 4-12 minutes. Read the manufacturer's instructions on the packet as a guide to cooking times. Drain the pasta thoroughly before tossing with the sauce of your choice.

DAY 5

150 CALORIES · MILK AND FAT ALLOWANCE

275ml (¹/₂ pint) skimmed milk
3 teaspoons low-fat spread or 1 teaspoon oil

— OR —

275ml (¹/₂ pint) semi-skimmed milk
2 teaspoons very low-fat spread
or ¹/₂ teaspoon oil

150 CALORIES · BREAKFASTS

30g (1oz) half-fat cheese, grilled on
20g (³/₄oz) slice toast
Grilled tomatoes

250 CALORIES · LIGHT MEALS

60g (2oz) lean ham or other lean cold meat or
85g (3oz) cooked kidney beans or chickpeas or
100g (3¹/₂oz) tuna in brine, drained
Green salad and tomatoes
3 crispbreads
1 peach or pear or 85g (3oz) grapes

— OR —

175g (6oz) potato, jacket baked or microwaved
150g (5oz) reduced-sugar and salt baked beans
Green salad

400 CALORIES · MAIN MEALS

Individual portion frozen fish in sauce
175g (6oz) potatoes mashed with milk
from allowance
85g (3oz) peas or mixed vegetables
150g (5oz) piece of fresh fruit

— OR —

Omelette made from 2 x size 4 eggs cooked
in a non-stick pan or microwaved
85g (3oz) peas
Grilled tomatoes
100g (3¹/₂oz) oven chips
1 kiwi fruit

— OR —

Grecian Style Baked Fish (see recipe page 78)
85g (3oz) peas or mixed vegetables
175g (6oz) potatoes mashed with milk from
allowance or 45g (1¹/₂oz) rice, boiled
1 kiwi fruit

100 CALORIES · EXTRAS

Anything up to 100 calories. All or part of this
allowance may be saved for another day.

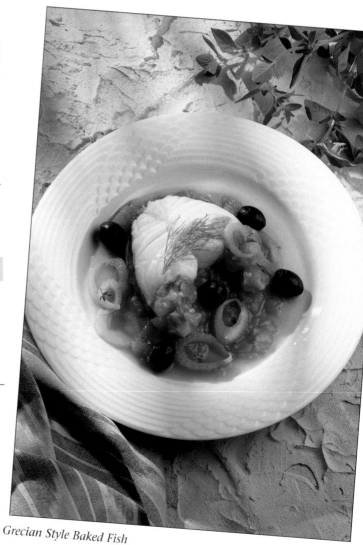

Grecian Style Baked Fish

DAY 6

150 CALORIES — MILK AND FAT ALLOWANCE

275ml (¹/₂ pint) skimmed milk
3 teaspoons low-fat spread or 1 teaspoon oil

— **OR** —

275ml (¹/₂ pint) semi-skimmed milk
2 teaspoons very low-fat spread
or ¹/₂ teaspoon oil

150 CALORIES — BREAKFASTS

175g (6oz) banana
1 diet yogurt

250 CALORIES — LIGHT MEALS

1 low-fat burger, grilled
1 burger bap
Salad garnish
1 satsuma

— **OR** —

1 take-away standard hamburger

— **OR** —

1 low-calorie Vegeburger (see recipe page 39)
Green salad and tomatoes
1 diet yogurt

400 CALORIES — MAIN MEALS

Any ready meal or vegetarian ready meal
up to 300 calories
200g (7oz) vegetables from low-calorie list
(see page 25)
1 diet yogurt or 1 diet fromage frais

— **OR** —

Sausage Hotpot (see recipe page 84)
75g (2¹/₂oz) green beans
75g (2¹/₂oz) cabbage
60g (2oz) ice cream

— **OR** —

Meal Out Choice (if going out)
Grilled or roast chicken quarter, skin removed,
or grilled plaice
Jacket or new potatoes, no butter unless fat
allowance has not been used
Green beans or salad, no dressing
*Tip: take your own oil-free dressing in a small
screwtop jar*

100 CALORIES — EXTRAS

Anything up to 100 calories.
All or part of this allowance may be saved
for another day.

Slimming tip: Weekends

Just because you have started your diet, you need not be afraid to eat out or entertain at weekends. The secret of surviving the weekend without ruining your slimming efforts is advance planning. If you have been saving up your Extras throughout the week, you will now have additional calories to spend, perhaps on a couple of glasses of wine, a cake or a delicious dessert – the choice is yours.

If you are eating out in a restaurant, learn how to make sensible choices on the menu (see page 96). Also, be aware of the hidden calories in many take-away meals if you are ordering food in; the photoguide on pages 100-101 will be helpful.

And if you do over-indulge at the weekend, all is not lost. Just go back on the diet again on Monday and stick with it, perhaps foregoing the Extras. Tomorrow is always another day, so just take it one day at a time and don't feel guilty. If you persevere, you can achieve your goal.

DAY 7

150 CALORIES — MILK AND FAT ALLOWANCE

275ml (¹/₂ pint) skimmed milk
3 teaspoons low-fat spread or 1 teaspoon oil

— OR —

275ml (¹/₂ pint) semi-skimmed milk
2 teaspoons very low-fat spread
or ¹/₂ teaspoon oil

150 CALORIES — BREAKFASTS

60g (2oz) lean trimmed back bacon, grilled
Grilled tomatoes or poached mushrooms
20g (³/₄oz) slice toast

— OR —

1 size 4 egg, poached
100g (3¹/₂ oz) reduced sugar and salt baked beans

250 CALORIES — LIGHT MEALS

60g (2oz) prawns or 4 seafood sticks
1 tablespoon low-calorie seafood dressing
Green salad
2 x 20g (³/₄oz) slices bread

Pineapple Fruit Salad

— OR —

250g (9oz) wedge of melon or 1 orange
1 pitta bread filled with salad
1 diet yogurt or 1 diet fromage frais

400 CALORIES — MAIN MEALS

60g (2oz) lean roast meat
3 tablespoons thin low-fat gravy
175g (6oz) potato, dry roast or jacket baked
75g (2¹/₂oz) cauliflower or broccoli
75g (2¹/₂oz) carrots
Pineapple Fruit Salad (see recipe page 76)
or 60g (2oz) ice cream

— OR —

Stuffed Courgettes (see recipe page 83)
60g (2oz) peas
60g (2oz) carrots
Pineapple Fruit Salad (see recipe page 76)
or 60g (2oz) ice cream

100 CALORIES — EXTRAS

Anything up to 100 calories. All or part of this
allowance may be saved for another day.

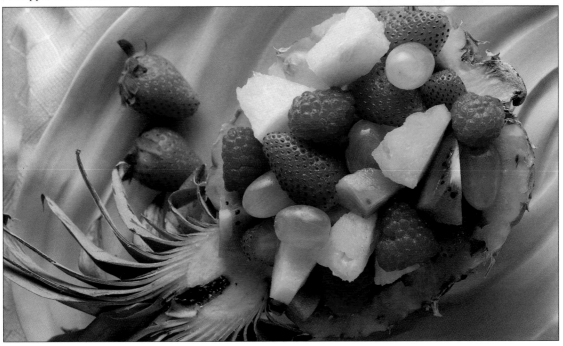

SNACKS

As you can see, the calories you consume in the form of snacks can vary considerably, so think carefully before you raid the fridge or reach for the biscuit tin.

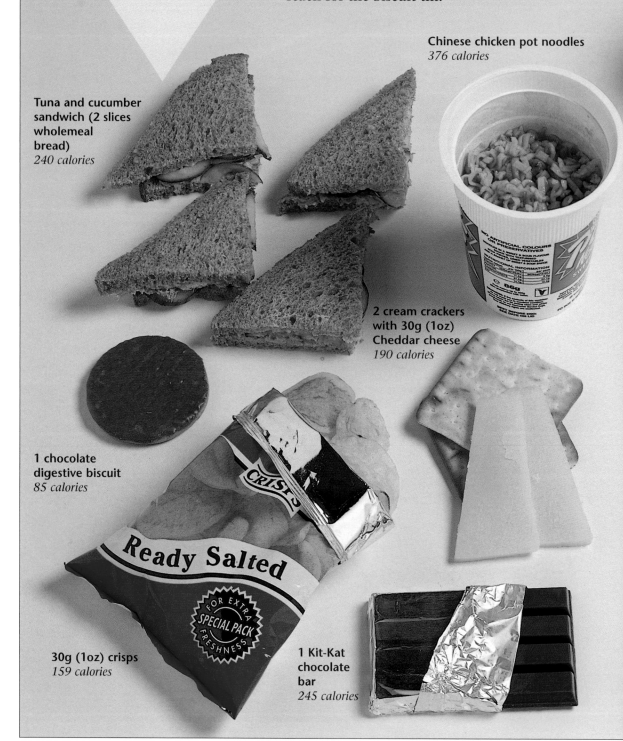

Chinese chicken pot noodles
376 calories

Tuna and cucumber sandwich (2 slices wholemeal bread)
240 calories

2 cream crackers with 30g (1oz) Cheddar cheese
190 calories

1 chocolate digestive biscuit
85 calories

30g (1oz) crisps
159 calories

1 Kit-Kat chocolate bar
245 calories

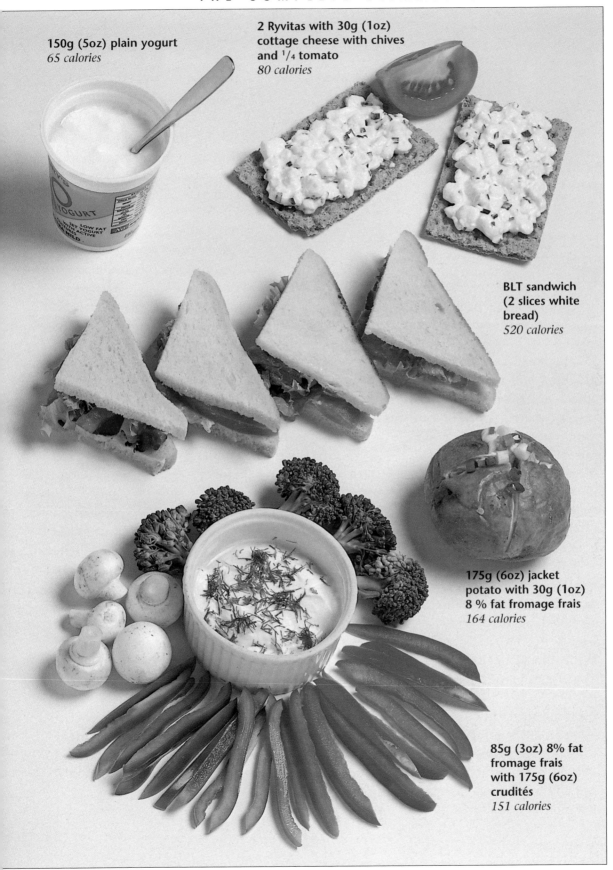

150g (5oz) plain yogurt
65 calories

2 Ryvitas with 30g (1oz) cottage cheese with chives and ¹/₄ tomato
80 calories

BLT sandwich (2 slices white bread)
520 calories

175g (6oz) jacket potato with 30g (1oz) 8 % fat fromage frais
164 calories

85g (3oz) 8% fat fromage frais with 175g (6oz) crudités
151 calories

1200 CALORIES DIET

10 steps to success

1 You should use this diet as your starting point if you are a woman and currently weigh between 10 and 12 stones.

2 You should choose one Breakfast, one Light Meal and one Main Meal each day from the suggestions that we have given you. These include vegetarian and packed lunch options.

3 You may eat your Breakfast, Light Meal and Main Meal in any order you wish, and at any time to suit your particular needs and lifestyle throughout the day. However, we recommend that meals are spaced fairly evenly throughout the day to prevent blood sugar levels dropping too low. This is when you are most likely to feel hungry and might be tempted to break your diet.

4 You should not skip meals. Make sure that you stick to the three meals per day.

5 Do not forget that every day you must have your Milk and Fat Allowance as set out on each page. You may use the Milk Allowance throughout the day in drinks, on cereal and in cooking. You may use the Fat Allowance on bread or crispbreads, in salad dressings and in cooking.

6 When following this diet, you may have 150 calories per day in the form of Extras to spread as you please These Extras are optional: you may use them each day OR save them up for a higher calorie item.

7 We have given you a complete week of meal ideas – you may choose one Breakfast, one Light Meal and one Main Meal from any of the seven daily menu plans prepared specially for this calorie level. You may also substitute a meal from the recipe section (see page 76) for any meal with a similar calorie count.

8 You can drop down to this calorie level if you have previously been consuming 1350 calories a day, or at a time when you need steady weight loss.

9 On the following pages, we have given you suggestions for the food that you need to eat to lose weight. However, there is more to losing weight than eating! If you are just starting to follow this diet, why not also start exercising too (see page 112)? If you have previously been following a different calorie level diet within this book, then you should continue to exercise and build up your level of activity slowly.

10 As you start to follow this calorie level, make a note of your weight at the start of the week. It is better if you do not weigh yourself again until the same time next week so that you can see the results of your efforts.

DAY 1

150 CALORIES MILK AND FAT ALLOWANCE

275ml (^{1}/$_2$ pint) skimmed milk
3 teaspoons low-fat spread or 1 teaspoon oil

OR

275ml (^{1}/$_2$ pint) semi-skimmed milk
2 teaspoons very low fat spread
or ^{1}/$_2$ teaspoon oil

200 CALORIES BREAKFASTS

45g (1^1/$_2$oz) non-sugar-coated cereal
150g (5oz) fresh fruit or 85g (3oz) banana
or 100g (3^1/$_2$oz) fruit canned in juice
or 115ml (4 fl oz) unsweetened citrus juice

300 CALORIES LIGHT MEALS

Sandwich made from
2 x 30g (1oz) slices bread
30g (1oz) half-fat cheese and 1 teaspoon pickle
or 30g (1oz) blue cheese and
finely chopped celery
1 kiwi fruit

OR

Lightly toast 2 x 30g (1oz) slices bread and fill
with lettuce, tomato, 60g (2oz) lean trimmed
back bacon, grilled, and 1 tablespoon
reduced-calorie salad cream
1 kiwi fruit

400 CALORIES MAIN MEALS

85g (3oz) skinless chicken breast, grilled or
oven-baked
175g (6oz) new potatoes
100g (3^1/$_2$oz) Brussels sprouts
100g (3^1/$_2$oz) carrots
1 peach or pear

OR

Curried Vegetables with rice (see recipe page 82)
125g carton low-fat natural yogurt mixed with
1 teaspoon honey

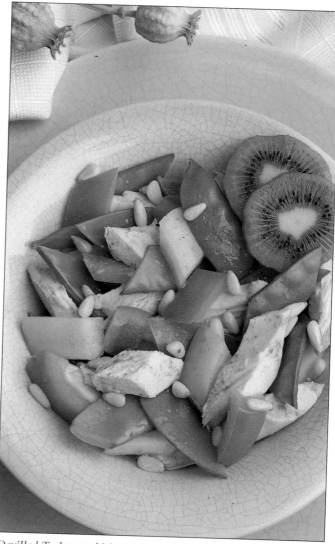

Devilled Turkey and Mange Tout Salad

OR

Devilled Turkey and Mange Tout Salad
(see recipe page 80)
150g (5oz) new potatoes
1 peach or pear

150 CALORIES EXTRAS

Anything up to 150 calories. All or part of this
allowance may be saved for another day.

150 CALORIES — MILK AND FAT ALLOWANCE

275ml (¹/₂ pint) skimmed milk
3 teaspoons low-fat spread or 1 teaspoon oil

— **OR** —

275ml (¹/₂ pint) semi-skimmed milk
2 teaspoons very low-fat spread
or ¹/₂ teaspoon oil

200 CALORIES — BREAKFASTS

2 x 30g (1oz) slices wholemeal toast
or 1 wholemeal English muffin
2 low-fat cheese triangles or 30g (1oz) low-fat
soft cheese
A scraping of yeast extract

300 CALORIES — LIGHT MEALS

60g (2oz) lean ham
or 1 cold chicken thigh, skin removed,
or 100g (3¹/₂oz) cooked kidney beans
Green salad and tomatoes
2 crispbreads
115g (4oz) banana
1 diet yogurt

— **OR** —

1 size 4 egg, poached
200g (7oz) reduced-sugar and salt spaghetti in
tomato sauce
1 orange
1 diet yogurt or 1 diet fromage frais

400 CALORIES — MAIN MEALS

Any ready meal or vegetarian ready meal up to
300 calories
200g (7oz) vegetables from low-calorie list
150g (5oz) piece fresh fruit

— **OR** —

Sausage Hotpot (see recipe page 84)
115g (4oz) potatoes, boiled or mashed with
milk from allowance
100g (3¹/₂oz) cabbage or green beans
1 kiwi fruit or satsuma

150 CALORIES — EXTRAS

Anything up to 150 calories. All or part of
this allowance may be saved for another day.

Sausage Hotpot

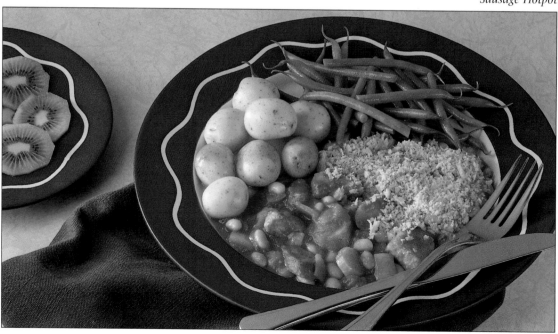

DAY 3

150 CALORIES — MILK AND FAT ALLOWANCE

275ml (^{1}/$_2$ pint) skimmed milk
3 teaspoons low-fat spread or 1 teaspoon oil

— OR —

275ml (^{1}/$_2$ pint) semi-skimmed milk
2 teaspoons very low-fat spread
or ^{1}/$_2$ teaspoon oil

200 CALORIES — BREAKFASTS

115ml (4fl oz) unsweetened citrus juice
or ^{1}/$_2$ grapefruit
1 size 4 egg, poached or boiled
30g (1oz) slice bread or toast

300 CALORIES — LIGHT MEALS

45g (1^1/$_2$oz) low-fat pâté or vegetarian pâté
3 crispbreads
2 tomatoes
1 'Twinpot' yogurt (approx. 100 calories) or
similar diet yogurt with fruit addition

— OR —

Any low-calorie soup up to 70 calories
30g (1oz) half-fat cheese
50g (1^3/$_4$oz) bread roll
1 satsuma

400 CALORIES — MAIN MEALS

85g (3oz) lean trimmed boneless pork chop or
gammon steak, grilled
1 ring of pineapple, grilled
85g (3oz) peas
Grilled tomatoes
175g (6oz) potato, jacket baked or microwaved
1 peach or pear or 250g (9oz) wedge of melon

— OR —

2 grilled vegetarian sausages
85g (3oz) peas
Grilled tomatoes
175g (6oz) potato, jacket baked or microwaved
1 peach or pear or 250g (9oz) wedge of melon

— OR —

1 low-calorie Vegeburger (see recipe below)
85g (3oz) peas
Grilled tomatoes
150g (5oz) potato, jacket baked or microwaved
1 diet yogurt or 1 diet fromage frais

100 CALORIES — EXTRAS

Anything up to 150 calories. You may save
part or all of this allowance for another day.

LOW-CALORIE VEGEBURGERS

These vegetarian-style burgers can be cooked inside on the grill or outside on the barbecue. For a more spicy version, add 1 tablespoon curry paste. This adds 10 calories per burger.

| 1 small onion, finely chopped |
| 1 garlic clove, crushed (optional) |
| 1 tablespoon oil |
| 175g (6oz) grated potato |
| 175g (6oz) grated carrot |
| 3 tablespoons chopped fresh herbs, e.g. parsley, coriander, chives |
| 115g (4oz) fresh breadcrumbs |

| 1 egg (size 3), beaten |
| salt and freshly ground black pepper |

1 Gently fry the onion and garlic in the oil until soft. Stir in the potato and carrot, and continue cooking for 5 minutes.

2 Transfer to a bowl and, when cool, add the herbs, breadcrumbs and seasoning. Bind with the beaten egg, and mould into 4 burgers.

3 Cook under a hot grill or on the barbecue for 10-15 minutes, turning half-way through the cooking.

Serves 4   *175 calories per burger*

150 CALORIES — MILK AND FAT ALLOWANCE

275ml (½ pint) skimmed milk
3 teaspoons low-fat spread or 1 teaspoon oil

OR

275ml (½ pint) semi-skimmed milk
2 teaspoons very low-fat spread
or ½ teaspoon oil

200 CALORIES — BREAKFASTS

115ml (4 fl oz) unsweetened citrus juice
45g (1½oz) muesli or 2 Weetabix

300 CALORIES — LIGHT MEALS

2 x 30g (1oz) slices bread
60g (2oz) prawns or drained tuna in brine
Lettuce and cucumber
1 tablespoon low-calorie seafood dressing
1 kiwi fruit and 1 satsuma

OR

2 x 30g (1oz) slices wholemeal toast
150g (5oz) reduced-sugar and salt baked beans
1 orange

400 CALORIES — MAIN MEALS

60g (2oz) pasta (dry weight), boiled, with 1 teaspoon
low-fat spread and 60g (2oz) lean diced ham
1 tablespoon grated parmesan cheese
Green side salad
250g (9oz) wedge of melon

OR

60g (2oz) pasta (dry weight), boiled, with
1 teaspoon low-fat spread and 45g (1½oz)
grated half-fat cheese
Green side salad
250g (9oz) wedge of melon

OR

Lasagne (see recipe right) and green salad

150 CALORIES — EXTRAS

Anything up to 150 calories. You may save part
or all of this allowance for another day.

LASAGNE

350g (12oz) lean minced beef

2 teaspoons oil

1 onion, finely chopped

1 garlic clove, crushed

1 carrot, diced

400g (14oz) canned chopped tomatoes

150ml (¼ pint) beef stock

1 tablespoon tomato paste

½ teaspoon dried basil or oregano

salt and freshly ground black pepper

115g (4oz) precooked lasagne

2 tablespoons grated Parmesan cheese

FOR THE WHITE SAUCE:

1 tablespoon low-fat spread

30g (1oz) seasoned plain flour

300ml (½ pint) skimmed milk

1 Cook the minced beef in its own fat in a non-stick pan until browned. Drain off the fat.

2 Heat the oil and sauté the onion, garlic and carrot until soft. Add the beef and tomatoes, and stir well. Add the stock, tomato paste, and herbs and bring to the boil. Simmer gently for 30-40 minutes. Season to taste.

3 Make the sauce: heat the fat and stir in the flour. Cook for 1-2 minutes, then stir in the milk. Bring to the boil, stirring until thick.

4 Pour half of the meat sauce into an ovenproof dish and cover with some lasagne sheets. Spoon half of the white sauce over the top and cover with the remaining meat sauce. Cover with the remaining lasagne, and top with the rest of the white sauce. Sprinkle with Parmesan and bake at 190°C/375°F/Gas Mark 5 for 30 minutes.

Serves 4 *385 calories per serving*

DAY 5

150 CALORIES MILK AND FAT ALLOWANCE

275ml (½ pint) skimmed milk
3 teaspoons low-fat spread or 1 teaspoon oil

— OR —

275ml (½ pint) semi-skimmed milk
2 teaspoons very low-fat spread
or ½ teaspoon oil

200 CALORIES BREAKFASTS

½ grapefruit or 250g (9oz) wedge of melon
30g (1oz) half fat cheese grilled on 30g (1oz)
slice toast

300 CALORIES LIGHT MEALS

Sandwich made from
2 x 30g (1oz) slices bread
45g (1½oz) lean corned beef
2 teaspoons pickle
1 kiwi fruit

— OR —

Sandwich made from
2 x 30g (1oz) slices bread
60g (2oz) firm tofu, sliced
1 tablespoon mango chutney or relish
1 kiwi fruit

— OR —

30g (1oz) lean trimmed back bacon, grilled
1 small low-fat sausage, grilled
60g (2oz) kidney, grilled
Grilled tomatoes
1 potato waffle, grilled
1 satsuma

400 CALORIES MAIN MEALS

175g (6oz) steamed white fish or smoked
haddock or cod
175g (6oz) potatoes, mashed with
milk from allowance
85g (3oz) peas
1 peach or orange

— OR —

2 size 4 eggs, poached
250g (9oz) spinach
175g (6oz) potatoes, mashed with
milk from allowance
1 peach or orange

— OR —

Mediterranean Fish Stew (see recipe page 80)
100g (3½oz) peas
1 peach or orange

150 CALORIES EXTRAS

Anything up to 150 calories. All or part of this
allowance may be saved for another day.

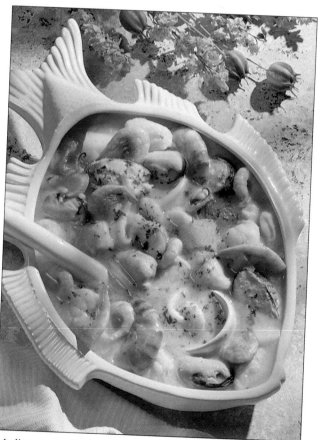

Mediterranean Fish Stew

DAY 6

150 CALORIES — MILK AND FAT ALLOWANCE

275ml (¹/₂ pint) skimmed milk
3 teaspoons low-fat spread or 1 teaspoon oil

— OR —

275ml (¹/₂ pint) semi-skimmed milk
2 teaspoons very low-fat spread
or ¹/₂ teaspoon oil

200 CALORIES — BREAKFASTS

115ml (4 fl oz) unsweetened citrus juice
50g (1³/₄oz) wholemeal or granary roll

300 CALORIES — LIGHT MEALS

1 tomato
1 frozen pizza slice
Large fresh salad
1 diet yogurt or 1 diet fromage frais

— OR —

1 burger bap filled with
2 grilled fish fingers
Lettuce and a squeeze of lemon juice
1 orange

400 CALORIES — MAIN MEALS

Any ready meal or vegetarian ready meal up to
300 calories
200g (7oz) vegetables from low-calorie list
1 diet yogurt or 1 diet fromage frais

— OR —

Tandoori Chicken (see recipe page 27)
100g (3¹/₂oz) green beans or green salad
30g (1oz) rice, boiled
60g (2oz) ice cream

— OR —

Meal Out or Takeaway Choice
1 serving prawn chop suey
3 tablespoons fried rice

150 CALORIES — EXTRAS

Anything up to 150 calories. All or part of this
allowance may be saved for another day.

Tandoori Chicken

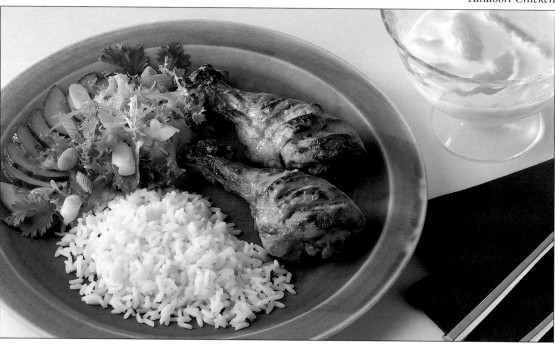

DAY 7

150 CALORIES — MILK AND FAT ALLOWANCE

275ml (¹/₂ pint) skimmed milk
3 teaspoons low-fat spread or 1 teaspoon oil

OR

275ml (¹/₂ pint) semi-skimmed milk
2 teaspoons very low-fat spread
or ¹/₂ teaspoon oil

200 CALORIES — BREAKFASTS

2 small low-fat sausages or 60g (2oz) lean
trimmed back bacon, grilled
Grilled tomatoes or poached mushrooms
30g (1oz) slice bread or toast

OR

30g (1oz) non-sugar-coated cereal
Grilled tomatoes or poached mushrooms
30g (1oz) slice bread or toast

300 CALORIES — LIGHT MEALS

115g (4oz) cottage cheese
175g (6oz) potato, jacket baked or microwaved
Green salad and tomatoes
150g (5oz) piece of fresh fruit

OR

1 size 4 egg, hard boiled
1 tablespoon low-calorie salad cream
Green salad and tomatoes
3 crispbreads or 30g (1oz) wholemeal bread
115g (4oz) banana

400 CALORIES — MAIN MEALS

60g (2oz) lean roast meat
3 tablespoon thin low-fat gravy
1 small frozen Yorkshire pudding
or 1 tablespoon stuffing or apple sauce
150g (5oz) potato, dry roast or jacket baked
75g (2¹/₂oz) Brussels sprouts or broccoli
75g (2¹/₂oz) carrots
1 meringue nest topped with 2 tablespoons
diet yogurt

OR

Cheesey Vegetable Bake (see recipe below)
75g (2¹/₂oz) peas
1 meringue nest topped with 2 tablespoon
diet yogurt

150 CALORIES — EXTRAS

Anything up to 150 calories. All or part of
this allowance may be saved for another day.

CHEESEY VEGETABLE BAKE

1 onion, chopped
1 garlic clove, crushed
350g (12oz) potatoes, peeled and thinly sliced
1 tablespoon oil
115g (4oz) mushrooms, sliced
1 red pepper, seeded and chopped
1 green pepper, seeded and chopped
400g (14oz) canned chopped tomatoes
275ml (¹/₂ pint) vegetable stock
1 tablespoon chopped herbs,
salt and freshly ground black pepper
150ml (¹/₄ pint) low-fat natural yogurt
85g (3oz) Mozzarella, sliced
85g (3oz) low-fat Cheddar cheese, grated
3 tablespoons fresh breadcrumbs

1 Sauté the onion, garlic and potatoes in the oil
for 5 minutes. Add the mushrooms, peppers
and tomatoes and cook gently for 5 minutes.

2 Add the stock, herbs and seasoning, and
bring to the boil. Reduce the heat and simmer
gently for about 20 minutes.

3 Transfer to a heatproof dish and spoon the
yogurt and cheeses over the top. Sprinkle
with breadcrumbs and pop under a
preheated grill for a few minutes until
bubbling and golden.

Serves 4   *300 calories per serving*

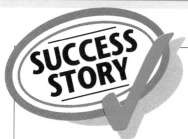

SUCCESS STORY

Jill Lawrence

All her life, Jill Lawrence had been plump, until she joined Slimmer Clubs UK and lost two-and-a-half stones. Jill says: "I never considered it a problem. I just thought I was big like the rest of my family. But when I got pregnant, the weight piled on –

I was eating for six, not two! Although I lost a little bit of weight after the birth, I couldn't keep it off, and so I joined my local Slimmer Club."

Jill thinks that the key to successful dieting is learning to eat in a healthy way. "No diet is plain sailing, and you need a lot of will-power, but it taught me to control my eating. I learnt that I could still enjoy chocolate and other high-calorie foods, but in moderation. I used to binge on them, but now I can put them away when I've had enough."

Jill has found that maintaining her weight is easy. "I just have slightly more of what I was eating on my diet, and intersperse it with treats. There is literally nothing that I don't eat. At home with my husband and young son, we eat a lot of pasta, rice and noodles. I tend to cook stir-fries and healthy meals with lots of vegetables that are really quick and easy to cook. I am more aware of what we eat now, and I always look for low-fat, healthy alternatives when I am out shopping."

Losing weight changed Jill's life. "It gave me back a sense of confidence and self-worth. I felt that I could do anything when I became a size 10. I was so pleased that I bought a whole new wardrobe of clothes, and gave away all the old big ones. I am now an Adviser for Slimmer Clubs UK so I've not only gained a new figure but a new job too!"

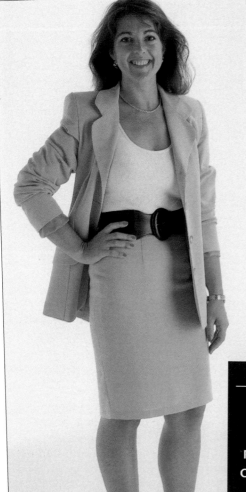

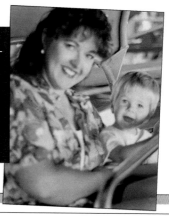

FACT FILE

Name: Jill Lawrence
Age: 30
Height: 5ft 3in
Past weight: 11st 10lbs
Current weight: 9st 2lbs

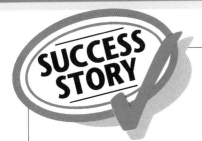

SUCCESS STORY

Sarah Bingham

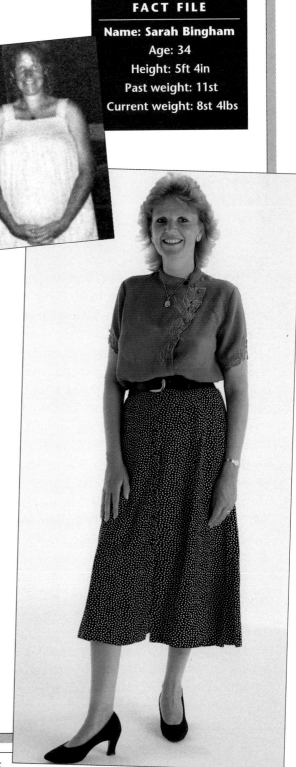

FACT FILE	
Name: Sarah Bingham	
Age: 34	
Height: 5ft 4in	
Past weight: 11st	
Current weight: 8st 4lbs	

Sarah had always been overweight and had tried 'every diet under the sun' before she joined Slimmer Clubs UK. "My weight ballooned up in my first pregnancy, and it was a shock when it didn't come off after the birth."

Eventually, Sarah joined her local Slimmer Club with a friend, and as a result she changed her eating habits and lost 2st 10lbs. She says: "I used to eat all the wrong things, but I learnt how to eat healthy foods, and I enjoyed them. When I got pregnant again I was much more sensible second time round and lost the weight easily afterwards.

"The secret of successful weight loss and maintenance for me has been to carry on going to class and having a regular weigh-in. When I was losing weight, I stuck rigidly to the diet all week, but now I can control my weight by being sensible Monday to Friday and then allowing myself more at weekends."

Sarah feeds the whole family healthy food. "We eat lots of rice, pasta, fresh vegetables, fish and white meat. We enjoy puddings, but we tend to have them just at weekends, not every day."

Sarah is featured in the exercise section (see page 112). Now working as an Area Manager for Slimmer Clubs UK, she finds it difficult to go to an exercise class regularly, but she does have a step at home and works-out two or three times a week. She also likes to go swimming and for walks with the family at weekends.

Her advice for slimmers is to set themselves a definite target. "This really motivated me and made me stick to the diet. As soon as I lost weight and grew out of clothes, I would throw them away, and when I got to my Gold Star Weight my husband treated me to a whole new wardrobe!"

1350 CALORIES DIET

10 steps to success

1 You should use this diet as your starting point if you are:
- A woman and currently weigh between 12st 1lb and 14st.
- Or if you are a man who is less than 5ft 5in tall.

2 You should choose one Breakfast, one Light Meal and one Main Meal every day from the suggestions that we have given you.

3 You may eat your Breakfast, Light Meal and Main Meal in any order and at any time to suit your particular needs throughout the day. We have included special options for vegetarians, and packed lunches for people who work and cannot cook in the middle of the day.

4 You should not skip meals. The diet has been carefully balanced to help you lose weight gradually and safely while providing all the essential nutrients that your body needs to stay healthy.

5 Do not forget that every day you must have your Milk and Fat Allowance as set out on each page. You may use the Milk Allowance throughout the day in drinks, on breakfast cereal and in cooking. You may use the Fat Allowance for spreading or cooking, and in salad dressings.

6 When following this diet you may have 250 calories each day in the form of Extras to spend as you please. These are optional: you may use them each day, either in one go or spread out throughout the day OR you may save them up for a higher calorie item.

7 We have given you a complete week of meal ideas. However, you may change the order as you wish and choose one Breakfast, one Light Meal and one Main Meal from any of the seven menu plans prepared specially for this calorie level. You may also substitute a meal from the recipe section (page 76) for any meal with a similar calorie count.

8 You can drop down to this calorie level if you have previously been consuming 1500 calories per day or at a time when you need steady weight loss.

9 On the following pages there are suggestions for the food that you need to eat to lose weight. However, there is more to losing weight than eating! If you are just starting to follow this diet, why not also start an exercise programme such as the work-out exercises on page 112? If you have previously been following a different calorie level diet within this book, then you should continue to exercise regularly and build up your level of activity slowly.

10 As you start to follow this calorie level diet, make a note of your weight at the beginning of the week. It is better if you do not weigh yourself again until the same time next week so that you can see the results of your efforts.

DAY 1

200 CALORIES — MILK AND FAT ALLOWANCE

425ml (¾ pint) skimmed milk
3 teaspoons low-fat spread or 1 teaspoon oil

— **OR** —

350ml (12 fl oz) semi-skimmed milk
2 teaspoons very low-fat spread
or ½ teaspoon oil

200 CALORIES — BREAKFASTS

45g (1½oz) non-sugar-coated cereal
150g (5oz) fresh fruit or 85g (3oz) banana
or 100g (3½oz) fruit canned in juice
or 115ml (4 fl oz) unsweetened citrus juice

300 CALORIES — LIGHT MEALS

1 "Pick'n'Mix" individual portion Babybel,
Port Salut or Edam or 30g (1oz) half-fat cheese
50g (1¾oz) French bread
2 tomatoes
1 kiwi fruit

— **OR** —

60g (2oz) lean ham or chicken or turkey
3 tablespoons sweetcorn
1 tablespoon reduced-calorie salad cream

150g (5oz) potato, jacket baked or microwaved
Green salad

400 CALORIES — MAIN MEALS

250g (9oz) chicken quarter (on bone),
skin removed
150g (5oz) new potatoes
75g (2½oz) green beans
75g (2½oz) carrots
1 satsuma

— **OR** —

Tortelloni Primavera (see recipe page 84)
1 diet yogurt or 1 diet fromage frais

— **OR** —

Sweet and Sour Pork (see recipe page 86)
1 diet yogurt

250 CALORIES — EXTRAS

Anything up to 250 calories. All or part of this
allowance may be saved for another day.

Tip: *¾ pint milk per day equals*
3 x 1 litre cartons per week

Tortelloni Primavera

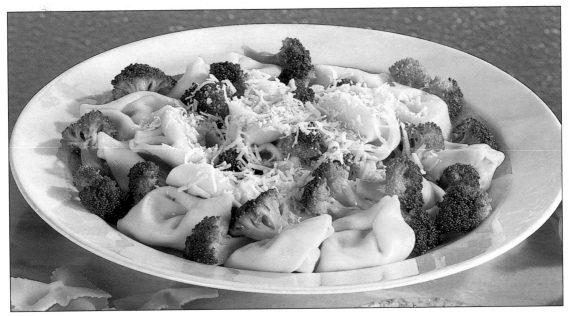

200 CALORIES — MILK AND FAT ALLOWANCE

425ml (¾ pint) skimmed milk
3 teaspoons low-fat spread or 1 teaspoon oil

OR

350ml (12 fl oz) semi-skimmed milk
2 teaspoons very low-fat spread
or ½ teaspoon oil

200 CALORIES — BREAKFASTS

½ grapefruit
2 x 30g (1oz) slices toast
Grilled tomatoes or poached mushrooms

300 CALORIES — LIGHT MEALS

115g (4oz) cottage cheese
4 crispbreads
Cucumber or tomato slices
2 x 150g (5oz) pieces fresh fruit

OR

100g (3½oz) tuna in brine, drained
Green salad and tomatoes
50g (1¾oz) wholemeal roll
1 apple

400 CALORIES — MAIN MEALS

Any ready meal or vegetarian ready meal up to
300 calories
200g (7oz) vegetables from low-calorie list
1 diet yogurt or 1 diet fromage frais

OR

Italian Hunter's Chicken (see recipe page 84)
115g (4oz) new potatoes
100g (3¹/₂oz) green beans

250 CALORIES — EXTRAS

Anything up to 250 calories. All or part of
this allowance may be saved for another day.

Italian Hunter's Chicken

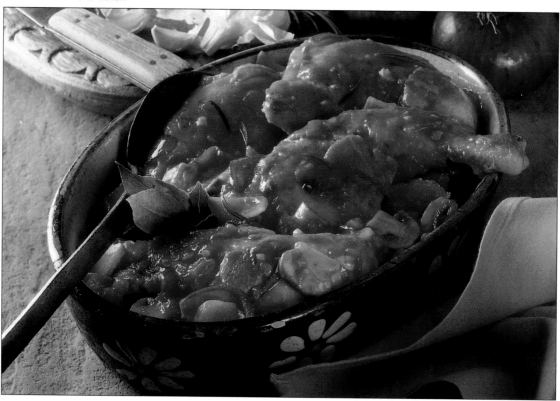

DAY 3

200 CALORIES MILK AND FAT ALLOWANCE

425ml (¾ pint) skimmed milk
3 teaspoons low-fat spread or 1 teaspoon oil

——— OR ———

350ml (12 fl oz) semi-skimmed milk
2 teaspoons very low-fat spread
or ½ teaspoon oil

200 CALORIES BREAKFASTS

115ml (4 fl oz) unsweetened citrus juice
1 size 4 egg, poached or boiled
30g (1oz) slice bread or toast

300 CALORIES LIGHT MEALS

60g (2oz) pack wafer thin ham, chicken or
turkey or 45g (1½oz) vegetarian pâté
2 tomatoes
Celery sticks
1 small packet lower fat crisps
1 'Twinpot' yogurt or similar diet yogurt
with fruit addition

——— OR ———

Soup made from 350g (12oz) diced vegetables
from low-calorie list simmered in 550ml
(1 pint) chicken or vegetable stock.
(Makes 2 bowls)
Top each bowl with 15g (½oz) grated
half-fat cheese
60g (2oz) ice cream

400 CALORIES MAIN MEALS

100g (3½oz) lean 'minute' steak, grilled
175g (6oz) potato, jacket baked or microwaved
100g (3½oz) peas or 60g (2oz) sweetcorn
Grilled tomatoes
250g (9oz) wedge of melon or 1 orange

——— OR ———

Vegetable Risotto (see recipe below)

——— OR ———

Low-calorie Beefburger (see recipe page 29)
75g (2½oz) peas
Grilled tomatoes
150g (5oz) potato, jacket baked or microwaved
250g (9oz) wedge of melon or 1 orange

250 CALORIES EXTRAS

Anything up to 250 calories. All or part of
this allowance may be saved for another day.

VEGETABLE RISOTTO

Ingredients
1 onion, chopped
2 garlic cloves, crushed
1 small red pepper, seeded and chopped
115g (4oz) mushrooms, sliced
1 teaspoons olive oil
200g (7oz) risotto rice
1 litre (1³/₄ pints) hot vegetable stock
250g (9oz) cooked kidney beans or 425g (15oz) can of kidney beans, rinsed and drained
salt and freshly ground black pepper
115g (4oz) grated half-fat Cheddar cheese

1 Sauté the onion, garlic, red pepper and mushrooms in the oil until tender. Add the rice and stir well over low heat, until the grains turn opaque.

2 Add some of the hot stock and bring to the boil. Reduce the heat to a simmer and cook gently, adding more stock as and when necessary, until it has all been absorbed and the rice is plump and tender.

3 Stir in the kidney beans and heat through gently. Season to taste with salt and pepper, and serve sprinkled with grated cheese.

Serves 4   *400 calories per serving*

DAY 4

200 CALORIES — MILK AND FAT ALLOWANCE

425ml (¾pint) skimmed milk
3 teaspoons low-fat spread or 1 teaspoon oil

— **OR** —

350ml (12 fl oz) semi-skimmed milk
2 teaspoons very low-fat spread
or ½ teaspoon oil

200 CALORIES — BREAKFASTS

1 Weetabix or Shredded Wheat
100g (3½oz) canned apricots in juice
30g (1oz) slice bread or toast
1 low-fat cheese triangle
or 2 teaspoons low-sugar jam

300 CALORIES — LIGHT MEALS

50g (1¾oz) wholemeal roll scraped with yeast
extract and filled with mustard and cress
115g (4oz) banana
1 diet yogurt or 1 diet fromage frais

— **OR** —

1 size 4 egg, hard boiled
1 tbsp low-calorie salad cream
Green salad and tomatoes
30g (1oz) wholemeal bread
150g (5oz) banana

400 CALORIES — MAIN MEALS

60g (2oz) extra lean minced beef, dry-fried or
microwaved and mixed with 100g (3½oz)
ready-made pasta sauce
60g (2oz) spaghetti or pasta shapes, boiled
1 teaspoon grated parmesan cheese
Green side salad

— **OR** —

Pasta with Tomato Sauce (see recipe page 86)
Green side salad
1 diet yogurt or 1 diet fromage frais

250 CALORIES — EXTRAS

Anything up to 250 calories. All or part of this
allowance may be saved for another day.

Pasta Main Meal

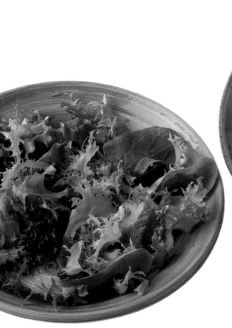
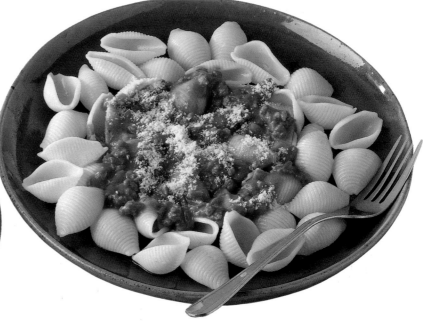

DAY 5

200 CALORIES — MILK AND FAT ALLOWANCE

425ml (¾ pint) skimmed milk
3 teaspoons low-fat spread or 1 teaspoon oil

OR

350ml (12 fl oz) semi-skimmed milk
2 teaspoons very low-fat spread
or ½ teaspoon oil

200 CALORIES — BREAKFASTS

Toasted sandwich made from
2 x 30g (1oz) slices bread
1 low-fat cheese slice
Sliced tomatoes or 15g (½oz) slice lean
vacuum-packed ham

300 CALORIES — LIGHT MEALS

Pitta bread filled with salad and 45g (1½oz)
lean corned beef or pastrami or 60g (2oz)
chicken or turkey

OR

2 x 30g (1oz) slices wholemeal bread
115g (4oz) banana, peeled and sliced

2 chopped dates and 2 chopped walnut halves

400 CALORIES — MAIN MEALS

200g (7oz) whole trout, grilled or 115g (4oz)
salmon steak, grilled or poached
150g (5oz) new potatoes
100g (3½oz) broccoli
250g (9oz) wedge of melon or 1 peach

OR

Omelette made from 2 size 4 eggs, cooked in a
non-stick pan or microwaved
150g (5oz) new potatoes
100g (3½oz) broccoli
100g (3½oz) peas or 60g (2oz) sweetcorn
250g (9oz) wedge of melon or 1 peach

OR

Fish Pie (see recipe below)
100g (3½oz) broccoli
250g (9oz) wedge of melon or 1 peach

250 CALORIES — EXTRAS

Anything up to 250 calories. All or part of
this allowance may be saved for another day.

FISH PIE

675g (1 ½lb) potatoes, cooked and mashed

275ml (½ pint) skimmed milk

450g (1lb) smoked haddock

1 tablespoon low-fat spread

1 small onion, chopped

1 leek, washed, trimmed and sliced

115g (4oz) mushrooms, sliced

1 tablespoon plain flour

60g (2oz) peeled cooked prawns

salt and pepper

1 tablespoon chopped parsley

1 Mix the potatoes with 3 tablespoons of the

milk. Season to taste with salt and pepper.

2 Poach the haddock in the remaining milk until cooked. Drain, reserving the milk, and flake into large pieces.

3 Heat the fat and sauté the onion and leek until soft. Add the mushrooms and cook gently for 3 minutes. Stir in the flour and cook over low heat for 1 minute. Add the reserved milk, a little at a time, stirring. Bring to the boil. Reduce the heat and add the prawns, seasoning, parsley and haddock.

4 Pour into an ovenproof dish and top with the potato. Bake in a preheated oven at 180°C/350°F/Gas Mark 4 for 20 minutes.

Serves 4   *310 calories per serving*

200 CALORIES — MILK AND FAT ALLOWANCE

425ml (¾ pint) skimmed milk
3 teaspoons low-fat spread or 1 teaspoon oil

— OR —

350ml (12 fl oz) semi-skimmed milk
2 teaspoons very low-fat spread
or ½ teaspoon oil

200 CALORIES — BREAKFASTS

115ml (4 fl oz) unsweetened citrus juice
60g (2oz) fruit and malt loaf or 1 small
wholemeal currant bun

300 CALORIES — LIGHT MEALS

French bread pizza made from
60g (2oz) French bread 'base' spread with 1
tablespoon tomato purée and pinch of oregano
Diced peppers or mushrooms
30g (1oz) sliced half-fat cheese
Bake in a moderate oven approx. 10 minutes

— OR —

1 large low-fat sausage, well grilled
1 finger roll
1 teaspoon mustard or ketchup
100g (3½oz) canned apricots in juice
30g (1oz) ice cream

400 CALORIES — MAIN MEALS

Any ready meal or vegetarian ready meal up to
300 calories
200g (7oz) vegetables from low-calorie list
1 diet yogurt or 1 diet fromage frais

— OR —

Spanish Rice (see recipe right)
1 kiwi fruit

— OR —

Meal Out or Takeaway choice
1 serving Chicken Tikka (not Masala) or
Tandoori Chicken

SPANISH RICE

1 tablespoon oil
1 medium onion, chopped
1 garlic clove, crushed
1 green chilli, seeded and chopped
225g (8oz) brown rice
550ml (1 pint) vegetable stock
400g (14oz) canned chopped tomatoes
½ red pepper, seeded and diced
½ green pepper, seeded and diced
115g (4oz) cooked peas (fresh or frozen)
salt and freshly ground black pepper
chopped parsley, to garnish
115g (4oz) half-fat cheese, grated

1 Heat the oil in a large non-stick frying pan and saute the onion and garlic until soft and translucent. Add the chilli and rice and cook for 2 minutes.

2 Add a little of the stock with the tomatoes and bring to the boil. Reduce the heat and then simmer gently, stirring occasionally and adding more stock as necessary, for 40 minutes. The rice is cooked when it is tender and has absorbed all the liquid.

3 Just before serving, stir in the peppers and peas. Season to taste, and serve sprinkled with parsley and grated half-fat cheese.

Serves 4   *365 calories per serving*

2 tablespoons boiled rice or 1 poppadum
Green salad or cucumber raita

250 CALORIES — EXTRAS

Anything up to 250 calories. All or part of this allowance may be saved for another day.

DAY 7

200 CALORIES MILK AND FAT ALLOWANCE

425ml (¾ pint) skimmed milk
3 teaspoons low-fat spread or 1 teaspoon oil

— OR —

350ml (12 fl oz) semi-skimmed milk
2 teaspoons very low-fat spread
or ½ teaspoon oil

200 CALORIES BREAKFASTS

1 size 4 egg, dry-fried or poached
30g (1oz) lean trimmed back bacon, grilled or
2 tablespoons reduced-sugar and
salt baked beans
30g (1oz) slice toast

— OR —

1 egg, size 4, dry-fried or poached
5 tablespoons reduced-sugar and salt baked beans
Grilled tomatoes

300 CALORIES LIGHT MEALS

Devilled Turkey and Mange tout Salad
(see recipe page 80)
2 crispbreads

— OR —

175g (6oz) potato, jacket baked or microwaved
30g (1oz) grated half-fat cheese
Green salad and tomatoes
1 diet yogurt or 1 diet fromage frais
1 satsuma

400 CALORIES MAIN MEALS

60g (2oz) lean roast meat
2 tablespoons thin low-fat gravy
1 small frozen Yorkshire pudding

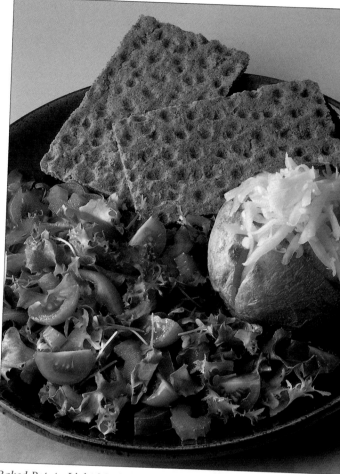

Baked Potato Light Meal

or 1 tablespoon stuffing or apple sauce
150g (5oz) potato, dry roast or jacket baked
75g (2½oz) Brussels sprouts or broccoli
75g (2½oz) carrots
100g (3½oz) canned fruit in juice
1 serving sugar-free jelly

— OR —

Cheesey Vegetable Bake (see recipe page 43)
100g (3½oz) peas
100g (3½oz) canned fruit in juice

250 CALORIES EXTRAS

Anything up to 250 calories. All or part of this
allowance may be saved for another day.

Slimming tip

Always check the labels on yogurts. They
should say either 'diet' or 'very low-fat' or
'virtually fat-free'. Those that say 'low-fat'
are often high in sugar and calories.

PACKED LUNCHES

Here are some slimming ideas for packed lunches that you can take to the office, school or college. They are all healthy and nutritious and low in calories. If you are buying ready-made sandwiches, read the labels to check the calorie counts – some are deceptively high.

Lunch box with 1 granary roll, carton of orange juice, salad, 30g (1oz) cheese, 30g (1oz) sweet pickle, 1 apple
380 calories

Egg mayonnaise sandwich (1 slice bread)
130 calories

2 tablespoons low-fat yogurt
16 calories

60g (2oz) fromage frais with mustard and vegetable crudités
104 calories

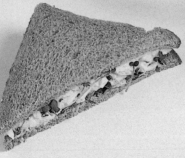

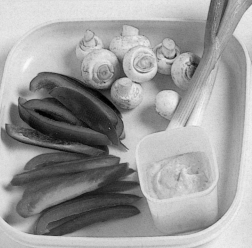

150g (5oz) fruit salad in juice
50 calories

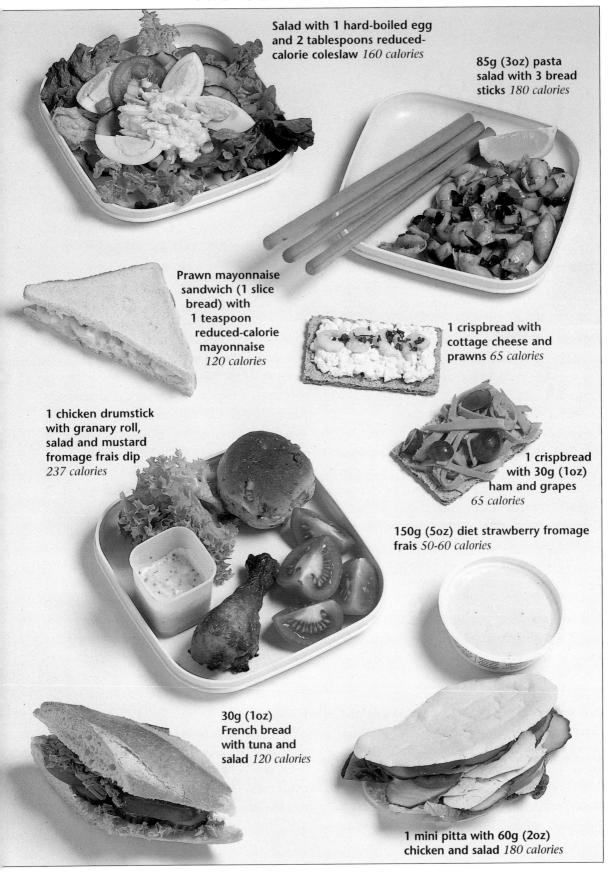

Salad with 1 hard-boiled egg and 2 tablespoons reduced-calorie coleslaw *160 calories*

85g (3oz) pasta salad with 3 bread sticks *180 calories*

Prawn mayonnaise sandwich (1 slice bread) with 1 teaspoon reduced-calorie mayonnaise *120 calories*

1 crispbread with cottage cheese and prawns *65 calories*

1 chicken drumstick with granary roll, salad and mustard fromage frais dip *237 calories*

1 crispbread with 30g (1oz) ham and grapes *65 calories*

150g (5oz) diet strawberry fromage frais *50-60 calories*

30g (1oz) French bread with tuna and salad *120 calories*

1 mini pitta with 60g (2oz) chicken and salad *180 calories*

1500 CALORIES DIET

10 steps to success

1 You should use this diet as your starting point if you are a woman and currently weigh between 14 stones 1 pound and 18 stones, or if you are a man currently weighing less than 15 stones. Girls between the ages of 10 and 18 years may also follow this diet after they have obtained the permission of their family doctor.

2 You should choose one Breakfast, one Light Meal and one Main Meal each day from the suggestions that we have given you. You will see that within each choice of meals there is a vegetarian option, and within the Light Meal selections there are meals that you can cook at home or ideas for packed lunches that you can take to work.

3 You may eat your Breakfast, Light Meal and Main Meal in any order you wish and at any time to suit your particular needs and routine throughout the day.

4 You should not skip meals, especially Breakfast. Make sure that you eat all three meals every day for a balanced diet.

5 Do not forget that every day you must have your Milk and Fat Allowance as set out on each page. You may use the Milk Allowance throughout the day in drinks, on cereal and in cooking. You may use the Fat Allowance for spreading on bread or crispbreads, or in salad dressings or for cooking.

6 When following this diet, you may have 250 calories per day to spend as you please. You may use them each day OR save them up for a higher calorie item.

7 We have given you a complete week of meal ideas but the diet plan is flexible. You may choose one Breakfast, one Light Meal and one Main Meal from any of the seven daily plans for this calorie level. You may also substitute a meal from the recipe section (see pages 76-93) for any meal with a similar calorie count.

8 You can drop down to this calorie level if you have previously been consuming 1650 calories a day, or at a time when you need steady weight loss.

9 On the following pages, we have given you suggestions for the food that you need to eat to lose weight, but there is more to losing weight than just eating! If you are just starting to follow this diet, why not start doing the work-out exercises (see page 112) or take up some other form of exercise, which will help burn up excess calories?

10 As you start to follow this calorie level, make a note of your weight at the start of the week. It is better if you do not weigh yourself again until the same time next week so that you can see the results of your efforts.

DAY 1

250 CALORIES — MILK AND FAT ALLOWANCE

550ml (1 pint) skimmed milk
3 teaspoons low-fat spread or 1 teaspoon oil

OR

500ml (18 fl oz) semi-skimmed milk
2 teaspoons very low-fat spread
or ½ teaspoon oil

200 CALORIES — BREAKFASTS

45g (1½oz) non-sugar-coated cereal
150g (5oz) fresh fruit or 85g (3oz) banana
or 115ml (4 fl oz) unsweetened citrus juice

300 CALORIES — LIGHT MEALS

50g (1¾oz) wholemeal or granary roll
30g (1oz) half-fat cheese
1 tomato
1 peach or pear

OR

3 fish fingers, grilled or 1 individual portion
frozen fish in parsley sauce
100g (3½oz) peas
Grilled tomatoes

30g (1oz) slice bread
1 satsuma

500 CALORIES — MAIN MEALS

250g (9oz) chicken quarter on the bone, skin
removed
175g (6oz) potato, jacket baked or microwaved
75g (2½oz) green beans
75g (2½oz) carrots
'Twinpot' yogurt or similar diet yogurt with
fruit addition

OR

Mediterranean Vegetable Pasta (see recipe page 89)
Green salad
125g carton low-fat natural yogurt mixed with
1 teaspoon honey

OR

Italian Stuffed Chicken (see recipe page 92)
100g (3½oz) broccoli
1 peach or pear

250 CALORIES — EXTRAS

Anything up to 250 calories. All or part of
this allowance may be saved for another day.

Mediterranean Vegetable Pasta

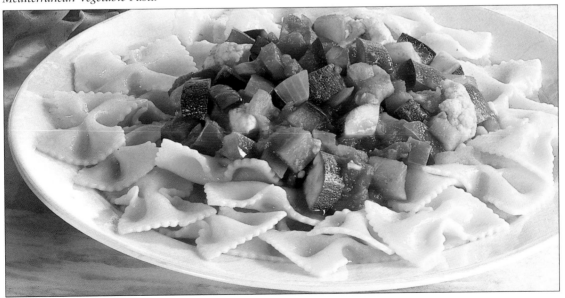

DAY 2

250 CALORIES — MILK AND FAT ALLOWANCE

550ml (1 pint) skimmed milk
3 teaspoons low-fat spread or 1 teaspoon oil

OR

500ml (18 fl oz) semi-skimmed milk
2 teaspoons very low-fat spread
or ½ teaspoon oil

200 CALORIES — BREAKFASTS

115ml (4 fl oz) unsweetened citrus juice
2 small oatcakes
30g (1oz) low-fat soft cheese or 60g (2oz)
cottage cheese

OR

115ml (4 fl oz) unsweetened citrus juice
45g (1½oz) porridge or instant porridge

300 CALORIES — LIGHT MEALS

1 size 4 egg, hard boiled
2 tomatoes
1 cereal bar up to 150 calories
1 orange

OR

100g (3½oz) tuna in brine, drained
or 85g (3oz) pilchards in tomato sauce
2 x 30g (1oz) slices bread or toast
Green salad and tomatoes
1 kiwi fruit

500 CALORIES — MAIN MEALS

Any ready meal or vegetarian ready meal up to
400 calories
200g (7oz) vegetables from low-calorie list
1 diet yogurt or 1 diet fromage frais

OR

Low-calorie Beefburger (see recipe page 29)
75g (2½oz) peas or mixed vegetables
Grilled tomatoes
150g (5oz) potato, jacket baked or microwaved
1 orange

250 CALORIES — EXTRAS

Anything up to 250 calories. You may save
part or all of this allowance for another day.

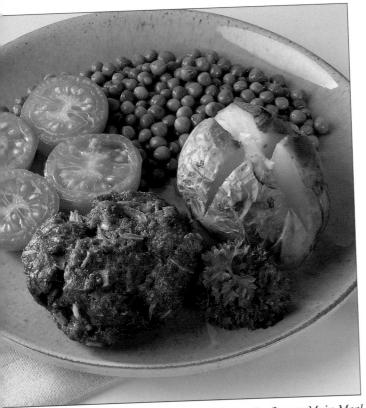

Beefburger Main Meal

DAY 3

250 CALORIES — MILK AND FAT ALLOWANCE

550ml (1 pint) skimmed milk
3 teaspoons low-fat spread or 1 teaspoon oil

— OR —

500ml (18 fl oz) semi-skimmed milk
2 teaspoons very low-fat spread or ½ teaspoon oil

200 CALORIES — BREAKFASTS

1 size 4 egg, poached or boiled
30g (1oz) slice bread or toast
115ml (4 fl oz) unsweetened citrus juice

300 CALORIES — LIGHT MEALS

3 crispbreads
45g (1½oz) low fat pâté or vegetarian pâté
Tomato or cucumber slices
1 orange
1 diet yogurt or 1 diet fromage frais

— OR —

50g (1¾oz) wholemeal or granary roll
1 orange
1 diet yogurt or 1 diet fromage frais

500 CALORIES — MAIN MEALS

85g (3oz) lean trimmed boneless pork chop or
gammon steak, grilled
85g (3oz) peas
Grilled tomatoes
175g (6oz) potato, jacket baked or microwaved
Orange Chocolate Pot (see recipe page 78) or
any pot dessert up to 165 calories

— OR —

Cauliflower Cheese (see recipe below)
85g (3oz) peas
Grilled tomatoes
150g (5oz) potato, jacket baked or microwaved
1 peach or pear or 85g (3oz) grapes

— OR —

Cheesey Vegetable Bake (see recipe page 43)
60g (2oz) ice cream
100g (3½oz) canned fruit in juice

250 CALORIES — EXTRAS

Anything up to 250 calories. You may save part
or all of this allowance for another day.

CAULIFLOWER CHEESE

| 1 medium cauliflower, broken into florets |
| 1 tablespoon margarine |
| 30g (1oz) plain flour |
| 275ml (1/2 pint) skimmed milk |
| 85g (3oz) half-fat cheese, grated |
| salt and pepper |
| 1/2 teaspoon Dijon mustard |

1 Cook the cauliflower in salted boiling water until it is just cooked and tender. Drain well and transfer to a heatproof dish.

2 Make the cheese sauce: melt the margarine in a small saucepan and stir in the flour to make a roux (paste). Remove from the heat and add the milk, a little at a time, stirring constantly until the sauce is blended and smooth.

3 Return the pan to the heat and bring to the boil, stirring. Add 60g (2oz) of the grated cheese and the seasoning and mustard. Reduce the heat and simmer gently for 2-3 minutes, stirring until the cheese melts.

4 Pour the sauce over the cauliflower and sprinkle with the remaining cheese. Put under a hot grill until hot and bubbling.

Serves 2   *360 calories per serving*

DAY 4

250 CALORIES — MILK AND FAT ALLOWANCE

550ml (1 pint) skimmed milk
3 teaspoons low-fat spread or 1 teaspoon oil

OR

500ml (18 fl oz) semi-skimmed milk
2 teaspoons very low-fat spread
or ½ teaspoon oil

200 CALORIES — BREAKFASTS

115ml (4 fl oz) unsweetened citrus juice
or ½ grapefruit
2 Weetabix or Shredded Wheat

300 CALORIES — LIGHT MEALS

1 pitta bread filled with salad and
45g (1½oz) lean ham, chicken or turkey or
60g (2oz) cooked kidney beans
1 kiwi fruit

OR

Dip of 100g (3½oz) fat-free natural fromage
frais mixed with a little tomato ketchup
250g (9oz) crudités (raw cauliflower, carrot,
celery, peppers, mushrooms, etc.)
150g (5oz) banana
30g (1oz) ice cream

500 CALORIES — MAIN MEALS

60g (2oz) extra lean minced beef, dry-fried or
microwaved and mixed with 100g (3½oz)
ready-made pasta sauce
60g (2oz) spaghetti or pasta shapes, boiled
1 tablespoon grated Parmesan cheese
Green side salad
1 diet yogurt
1 satsuma

OR

Quorn Spaghetti Bolognese
(see recipe page 80)
Green side salad
115g (4oz) banana plus
60g (2oz) ice cream

OR

Chilli Con Carne with rice (see recipe page 90)
Green side salad
1 satsuma

250 CALORIES — EXTRAS

Anything up to 250 calories. You may save
part or all of this allowance for another day.

Quorn Spaghetti Bolognese

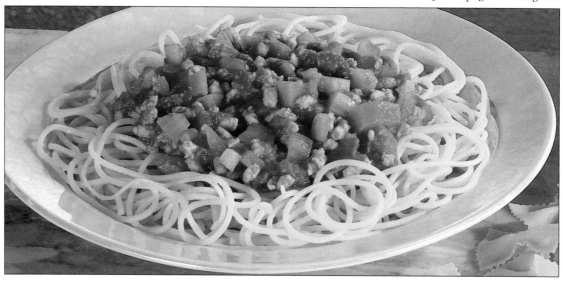

DAY 5

250 CALORIES — MILK AND FAT ALLOWANCE

550ml (1 pint) skimmed milk
3 teaspoons low-fat spread or 1 teaspoon oil

— OR —

500ml (18 fl oz) semi-skimmed milk
2 teaspoons very low-fat spread
or ½ teaspoon oil

200 CALORIES — BREAKFASTS

1 diet yogurt or diet fromage frais
2 x 30g (1oz) slices toast
Grilled tomatoes or poached mushrooms

300 CALORIES — LIGHT MEALS

50g (1¾oz) wholemeal or granary roll filled
with 30g (1oz) lean corned beef and
1 tablespoon reduced-calorie coleslaw
1 orange

— OR —

115g (4oz) cottage cheese with chives
175g (6oz) potato, jacket baked or microwaved
or 50g (1¾oz) wholemeal or granary roll
Green salad and tomatoes
1 kiwi fruit

500 CALORIES — MAIN MEALS

100g (3½oz) portion lower-fat oven-bake fish
100g (3½oz) oven chips
100g (3½oz) peas
1 diet yogurt
150g (5oz) piece of fresh fruit

— OR —

Omelette made from 2 size 4 eggs, cooked in a
non-stick pan or microwave
150g (5oz) new potatoes
100g (3½oz) mixed vegetables
150g (5oz) low-fat rice pudding
200g (7oz) canned apricots in juice

— OR —

Fish Pie (see recipe page 51)
100g (3½oz) broccoli
100g (3½oz) mixed vegetables
200g (7oz) canned apricots in juice

250 CALORIES — EXTRAS

Anything up to 250 calories. All or part of this
allowance may be saved for another day.

Slimming tip: Extras

Every day, you are allocated an 'Extras' allowance – on this diet, up to 250 calories. The temptation is to blow all this on your favourite chocolate bar or weakness. However, it's not really a sensible idea to spend all your 'Extras' on treat foods – after all, these are probably the foods that made you put on weight in the first place.

If you want to get slim and stay that way, then you need to change your eating habits permanently. Most successful slimmers testify that as a result of our diet, they discovered how delicious fruit and vegetables can be and now actually enjoy eating healthier food.

So keep sugary and high-fat items as occasional treats, and not as a regular indulgence. Remember that the less you have, the less you will crave for them, and the better your chances of sticking to your diet and achieving long-term success.

250 CALORIES — MILK AND FAT ALLOWANCE

550ml (1 pint) skimmed milk
3 teaspoons low-fat spread or 1 teaspoon oil

OR

500ml (18 fl oz) semi-skimmed milk
2 teaspoons very low-fat spread
or ½ teaspoon oil

200 CALORIES — BREAKFASTS

2 toasted crumpets
2 teaspoons low-sugar jam

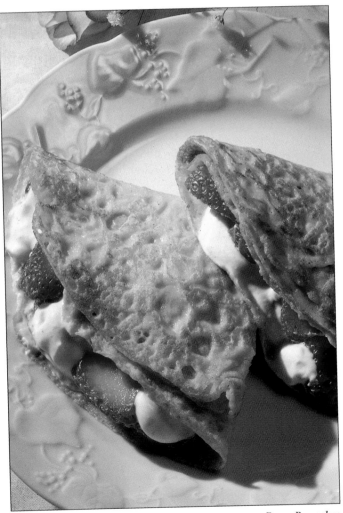

Berry Pancakes

300 CALORIES — LIGHT MEALS

1 frozen pizza slice or 5-inch frozen pizza
up to 250 calories
Green salad
1 kiwi fruit

OR

1 low-fat burger, grilled
1 burger bun
1 teaspoon ketchup, mustard or relish
Salad garnish
1 orange

500 CALORIES — MAIN MEALS

Any ready meal up to 400 calories
200g (7oz) vegetables from low-calorie list
1 diet yogurt or 1 diet fromage frais

OR

Sausage Hotpot (see recipe page 84)
Green side salad
Berry Pancakes (see recipe page 77)
or 150g (5oz) banana with 60g (2oz) ice cream

OR

Meal Out or Takeaway Choice
150g (5oz) grilled steak
Jacket potato (no butter)
Green beans or salad (no dressing)
Fruit salad

OR

2 pieces Southern Fried Chicken
Regular Fries
No Extras calories if you choose this!

250 CALORIES — EXTRAS

Anything up to 250 calories. All or part of this
allowance may be saved for another day.

DAY 7

250 CALORIES — MILK AND FAT ALLOWANCE

550ml (1 pint) skimmed milk
3 teaspoons low-fat spread or 1 teaspoon oil

— OR —

500ml (18 fl oz) semi-skimmed milk
2 teaspoons very low-fat spread
or ½ teaspoon oil

200 CALORIES — BREAKFASTS

1 size 4 egg, scrambled with milk and spread
from allowance
30g (1oz) lean vacuum packed ham
Grilled tomato
30g (1oz) slice wholemeal toast

— OR —

Vegetarians may replace the ham with poached
mushrooms or 1 tablespoon soya 'bacon bits'

300 CALORIES — LIGHT MEALS

250g (9oz) wedge of melon, peeled and diced
60g (2oz) prawns or 3 seafood sticks, diced
Lettuce leaves
1 or 2 teaspoon oil-free dressing
30g (1oz) slice wholemeal bread
1 'Twinpot' diet yogurt

— OR —

150g (5oz) reduced-sugar and salt baked beans
2 x 30g (1oz) slices wholemeal toast or 150g
(5oz) potato, jacket baked or microwaved
Green salad
1 diet yogurt or 1 diet fromage frais

500 CALORIES — MAIN MEALS

85g (3oz) lean roast meat
3 tablespoon thin low-fat gravy
1 small frozen Yorkshire pudding or
1 tablespoon stuffing or apple sauce
150g (5oz) potato, dry roast or jacket baked
75g (2½oz) Brussels sprouts or broccoli
75g (2½oz) carrots
200g (7oz) baked apple stuffed with
15g (½oz) raisins or 2 dates

— OR —

Spanish Rice (see recipe page 52)
225g (8oz) baked apple stuffed with
15g (½oz) raisins or 2 dates

— OR —

or Stir-fried Thai Beef with noodles
(see recipe page 90)
1 satsuma

250 CALORIES — EXTRAS

Anything up to 250 calories. All or part of this
allowance may be saved for another day.

Slimming tip

When you're entertaining, don't feel
obliged to serve your guests large high-
calorie meals. You can still create a
special meal with healthy, low-calorie
food and simple, top-quality
ingredients. Look through the recipes
in this book for some delicious ideas.

BREAKFASTS

Breakfast is an important meal when you are on a diet, yet breakfasts can vary considerably in calorie content as shown by the selection here. Try to avoid buttery croissants and pastries which are extremely high in calories.

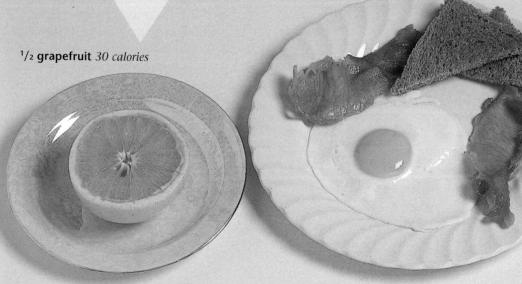

¹/₂ **grapefruit** *30 calories*

1 fried egg, 2 rashers grilled back bacon with 1 slice toast *275 calories*

30g (1oz) cornflakes *110 calories*

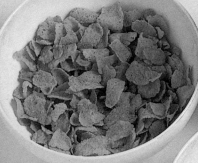

115ml (4 fl oz) semi-skimmed milk *52 calories*

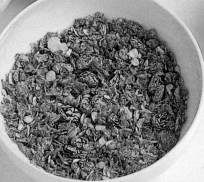

30g (1oz) muesli *115 calories*

100ml (3 ¹/₂ fl oz) unsweetened orange juice *40 calories*

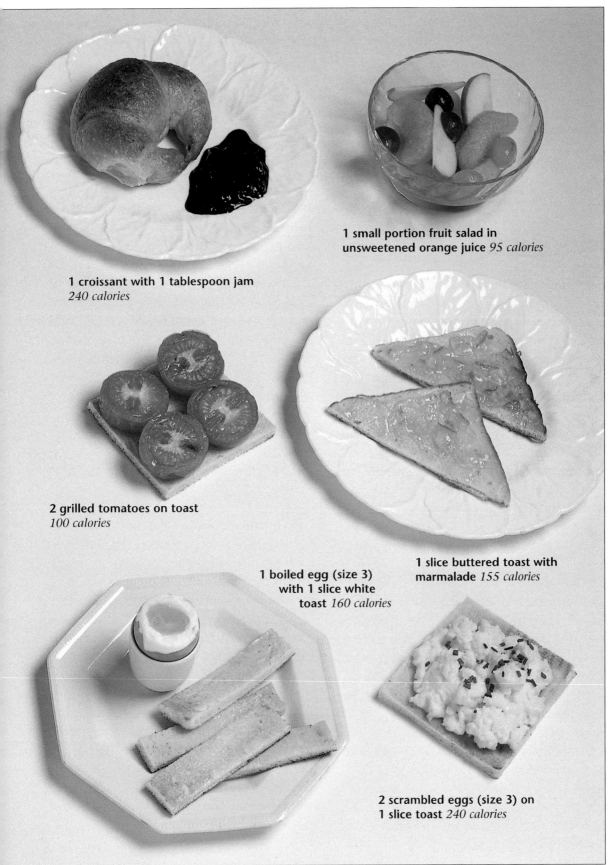

1 small portion fruit salad in unsweetened orange juice *95 calories*

1 croissant with 1 tablespoon jam *240 calories*

2 grilled tomatoes on toast *100 calories*

1 slice buttered toast with marmalade *155 calories*

1 boiled egg (size 3) with 1 slice white toast *160 calories*

2 scrambled eggs (size 3) on 1 slice toast *240 calories*

1650 CALORIES DIET

10 steps to success

1 You should use this diet as your starting point if you are a woman and currently weigh over 18 stones, or if you are a man currently weighing more than 15 stones. Boys and girls between the ages of 10 and 18 years may also follow this diet after they have obtained the permission of their doctor.

2 You should choose one Breakfast, one Light Meal and one Main Meal each day from the suggestions given. Within each choice of meals, there is a vegetarian option, and within the Light Meal selections there are meals that you can cook at home or ideas for packed lunches that you can take to work.

3 You may eat your Breakfast, Light Meal and Main Meal in any order and at any time to suit your particular needs throughout the day. However, we recommend that meals are spaced fairly evenly to prevent blood sugar levels dropping too low. This is when you are most likely to feel hungry and might be tempted to break your diet.

4 You should not skip meals. Make sure that you stick to the three meals a day.

5 Do not forget that every day you must also have your Milk and Fat Allowance as set out on each page. You may use the Milk Allowance throughout the day in drinks and on cereal and in cooking. You may use the Fat Allowance for spreading on bread, crisp-breads, baked potatoes and in salad dressings.

6 When following this diet you may have 300 calories per day to spend as you please. You may use them each day OR save them up for a higher calorie item.

7 We have given you a complete week of meal ideas but the diet plan is flexible. You may choose one Breakfast, one Light Meal and one Main Meal from any of the seven daily plans for this calorie level. You may also substitute a meal from the recipe section for any meal with a similar calorie count.

8 You may change to this diet if you have previously been following the 1500 calorie diet but have now embarked upon strenuous exercise.

9 On the following pages, we have given you suggestions for the food that you need to lose weight, but there is more to losing weight than just eating. Why not start doing the work-out exercises (see page 112) or take up some other form of exercise?. If you have previously been following a different calorie level diet within this book, you should continue to exercise regularly and build slowly.

10 As you start to follow this calorie level, make a note of your weight at the start of the week. It is better if you do not weigh yourself again until the same time next week, wearing the same clothes, so that you can see the results of your efforts.

DAY 1

250 CALORIES — MILK AND FAT ALLOWANCE

550ml (1 pint) skimmed milk
3 teaspoons low-fat spread or 1 teaspoon oil

— OR —

500ml (18 fl oz) semi-skimmed milk
2 teaspoons very low-fat spread
or ½ teaspoon oil

300 CALORIES — BREAKFASTS

115ml (4 fl oz) unsweetened citrus juice
2 Weetabix or Shredded Wheat or 50g (1¾oz)
wholemeal or granary roll
150g (5oz) banana or 200g (7oz) canned
apricots in juice

300 CALORIES — LIGHT MEALS

Sandwich made from
2 x 30g (1oz) slices bread
60g (2oz) lean ham
or 45g (1½oz) vegetarian pâté
Salad garnish
1 diet yogurt or 1 peach or pear

— OR —

Individual portion frozen fish in sauce
100g (3½oz) peas
30g (1oz) slice wholemeal bread
1 satsuma

500 CALORIES — MAIN MEALS

1 Breaded Turkey Escalope or Southern Fried
Chicken, up to 275 calories,
ovenbaked or grilled
175g (6oz) potato, jacket baked or
microwaved
100g (3½oz) green beans
100g (3½oz) carrots
250g (9oz) wedge of melon or
85g (3oz) grapes

— OR —

Butter bean Bake (see recipe page 86)
Green salad
100g (3½oz) canned apricots in natural juice
with 60g (2oz) ice-cream

— OR —

Chicken with Peanut Satay Sauce and rice
(see recipe page 90)
Green salad

300 CALORIES — EXTRAS

Anything up to 300 calories. All or part of this
allowance may be saved for another day.

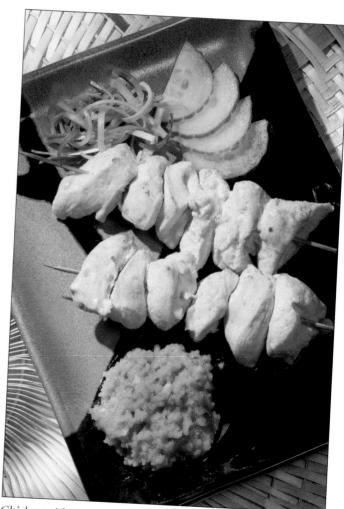

Chicken with Peanut Satay Sauce

DAY 2

250 CALORIES — MILK AND FAT ALLOWANCE

550ml (1 pint) skimmed milk
3 teaspoons low-fat spread or 1 teaspoon oil

— OR —

500ml (18 fl oz) semi-skimmed milk
2 teaspoons very low-fat spread
or ½ teaspoon oil

300 CALORIES — BREAKFASTS

½ grapefruit or 100g (3½oz) canned grapefruit
segments in juice
3 small low-fat sausages, grilled
Grilled tomatoes
30g (1oz) slice bread or toast

— OR —

1 toasted muffin or 1 small bagel,
1 egg, scrambled in non-stick pan
115ml (4 fl oz) unsweetened citrus juice

300 CALORIES — LIGHT MEALS

30g (1oz) half-fat cheese
150g (5oz) apple
15g (½oz) raisins
2 small digestive biscuits or
50g (1¾oz) wholemeal roll

— OR —

85g (3oz) pilchards on
2 x 30g (1oz) slices toast
1 orange

500 CALORIES — MAIN MEALS

Any ready meal or vegetarian ready meal up to
400 calories
200g (7oz) vegetables from low-calorie list
1 diet yogurt or 1 diet fromage frais

— OR —

115g (4oz) liver and 30g (1oz) sliced onions
braised in 150ml (¼pint) gravy made from
gravy powder
175g (6oz) potato mashed with milk from
allowance

PESTO SPAGHETTI

375g (12oz) spaghetti

115g (4oz) button mushrooms, halved

2 teaspoons oil

4 tablespoons ready-made pesto sauce

150ml (5 fl oz) low-fat natural yogurt

salt and freshly ground black pepper

2 tablespoons grated Parmesan cheese

1 Cook the spaghetti in boiling lightly salted water until tender. Drain well.

2 Meanwhile, sauté the mushrooms in the oil until golden. Mix with the pesto sauce and yogurt into the cooked spaghetti, and season to taste. Serve sprinkled with Parmesan cheese.

Serves 4   420 calories per serving

Note: You can buy ready-made pesto sauce in most supermarkets now as well as in Italian delicatessens. It can be purchased in jars, or freshly made in tubs. Because it is very oily and high in calories, it must be used sparingly – delicious though it is! Keep a jar in the refrigerator and blend a tablespoonful with low-fat yogurt or fromage frais for mixing with pasta, or as a topping for baked potatoes, or to serve with grilled chicken or fish.

100g (3½oz) cabbage
75g (2½oz) carrots
1 diet yogurt or 1 diet fromage frais

— OR —

Pesto Spaghetti (see recipe above)
Green salad and tomatoes
1 orange or 225g (8oz) wedge of melon

300 CALORIES — EXTRAS

Anything up to 300 calories. You may save part
or all of this allowance for another day.

DAY 3

250 CALORIES — MILK AND FAT ALLOWANCE

550ml (1 pint) skimmed milk
3 teaspoons low-fat spread or 1 teaspoon oil

— **OR** —

500ml (18 fl oz) semi-skimmed milk
2 teaspoons very low-fat spread
or ½ teaspoon oil

300 CALORIES — BREAKFASTS

115ml (4 fl oz) unsweetened citrus juice
1 size 4 egg, boiled or poached
2 x 30g (1oz) slices bread or toast
2 teaspoons low-sugar jam or 1 teaspoon honey

300 CALORIES — LIGHT MEALS

45g (1½oz) low-fat pâté
or 3 teaspoons peanut butter
3 crispbreads
2 tomatoes
1 diet yogurt or 1 diet fromage frais
1 kiwi fruit

— **OR** —

Curried Vegetables (see recipe page 82)
with rice

500 CALORIES — MAIN MEALS

115g (4oz) lean 'minute' steak or well trimmed
lamb chop, grilled
175g (6oz) potato, jacket baked or microwaved
100g (3½oz) peas or mixed vegetables
Grilled tomatoes
100g (3½oz) canned fruit in juice
30g (1oz) ice cream

— **OR** —

Vegetable Crêpes (see recipe page 89)
Green salad
100g (3½oz) canned fruit in juice
1 diet yogurt or 1 diet fromage frais

— **OR** —

Sausage Hotpot (see recipe page 84)
175g (6oz) potatoes, boiled or mashed with
milk from allowance
100g (3½oz) Brussels sprouts
250g (9oz) wedge of melon or 85g (3oz) grapes

300 CALORIES — EXTRAS

Anything up to 300 calories. All or part of this
allowance may be saved for another day.

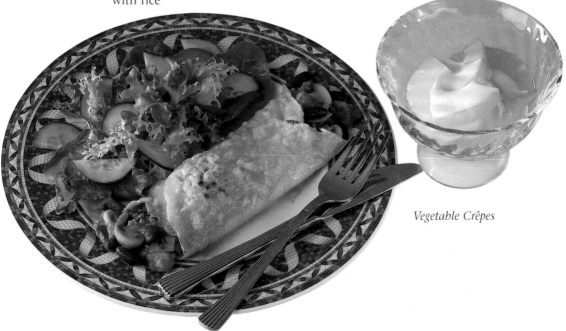

Vegetable Crêpes

DAY 4

250 CALORIES — MILK AND FAT ALLOWANCE

550ml (1 pint) skimmed milk
3 teaspoons low-fat spread or 1 teaspoon oil

— **OR** —

500ml (18 fl oz) semi-skimmed milk
2 teaspoons very low-fat spread
or ½ teaspoon oil

300 CALORIES — BREAKFASTS

½ grapefruit or 100g (3½oz) canned grapefruit
segments in juice
45g (1½oz) non-sugar-coated cereal
30g (1oz) slice toast
2 teaspoon low-sugar jam
or 1 low-fat cheese triangle

300 CALORIES — LIGHT MEALS

50g (1¾oz) bap filled with
1 size 4 egg, hard boiled and sliced
1 tablespoon low-calorie salad cream
Mustard and cress
1 orange

— **OR** —

100g (3½oz) tuna in brine, drained
or 85g (3oz) prawns
Green salad and tomatoes
30g (1oz) slice wholemeal bread
100g (3½oz) canned fruit in juice
30g (1oz) ice cream

500 CALORIES — MAIN MEALS

Chilli con Carne (see recipe page 90)
Green side salad

— **OR** —

Vegetable Chilli (see recipe page 93)
60g (2oz) brown rice, boiled
Green side salad
125g carton natural low fat yogurt

— **OR** —

Spaghetti Bolognese (see recipe page 93)
Green side salad
1 satsuma

300 CALORIES — EXTRAS

Anything up to 300 calories. You may save part
or all of this allowance for another day.

Spaghetti Bolognese

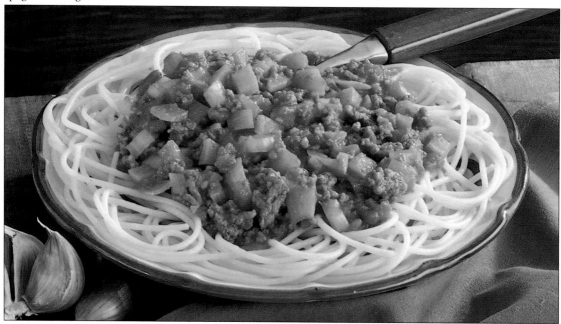

DAY 5

250 CALORIES — MILK AND FAT ALLOWANCE

550ml (1 pint) skimmed milk
3 teaspoons low-fat spread or 1 teaspoon oil

— **OR** —

500ml (18 fl oz) semi-skimmed milk
2 teaspoons very low-fat spread
or ½ teaspoon oil

300 CALORIES — BREAKFASTS

60g (2oz) half-fat cheese grilled on
2 x 30g (1oz) slices wholemeal toast

300 CALORIES — LIGHT MEALS

200g (7oz) reduced-sugar and salt baked beans
eaten hot or cold, or 150g (5oz) cooked kidney
beans or other cooked beans
50g (1¾oz) wholemeal roll
1 satsuma

— **OR** —

60g (2oz) lean corned beef or pastrami
Green salad and tomatoes
30g (1oz) slice bread
1 satsuma
1 diet yogurt or 1 diet fromage frais

500 CALORIES — MAIN MEALS

200g (7oz) white fish, steamed
or 115g (4oz) oily fish (e.g. mackerel), grilled
175g (6oz) potato, boiled or mashed with milk
from allowance
100g (3½oz) peas or mixed vegetables
150g (5oz) banana

— **OR** —

Omelette made from 2 size 4 eggs, cooked in a
non-stick pan or microwaved
Poached mushrooms
100g (3½oz) peas or mixed vegetables
100g (3½oz) oven chips
150g (5oz) banana

— **OR** —

Seafood Risotto (see recipe page 88)
60g (2oz) peas
Pineapple Fruit Salad (see recipe page 76)

300 CALORIES — EXTRAS

Anything up to 300 calories. All or part of this
allowance may be saved for another day.

Slimming tip: Low-calorie shopping

When you are pushing your trolley up and down the aisles of your local supermarket, always choose low-fat and low-calorie foods whenever possible. Remember that vegetables are very low in calories and are always a sensible and healthy purchase when you are dieting. Fresh fruit makes a slimming alternative to creamy desserts and puddings, so why not treat yourself to some exotic varieties as well as your usual orange, apples and bananas? Here are some more ideas for low-calorie alternatives:

- Very low-fat cottage cheese
- Skimmed milk
- Diet yogurt
- Canned fruit in natural juice
- Reduced-sugar canned beans
- Canned tuna in brine, not oil
- Sardines in tomato sauce, not oil
- Half-fat cheese
- Low-calorie mayonnaise
- Low-fat salad dressings
- Reduced-calorie ice cream and sorbets
- Low-fat spreads
- Virtually fat-free fromage frais
- Reduced-sugar jam
- Artificial sweeteners
- Unsweetened fruit juice
- Low-calorie mixers and diet drinks
- Non-sugar coated cereals

250 CALORIES — MILK AND FAT ALLOWANCE

550ml (1 pint) skimmed milk
3 teaspoons low-fat spread or 1 teaspoon oil

— **OR** —

500ml (18 fl oz) semi-skimmed milk
2 teaspoons very low-fat spread
or ½ teaspoon oil

300 CALORIES — BREAKFASTS

1 large bagel
45g (1½oz) low-fat soft cheese

300 CALORIES — LIGHT MEALS

Leek and Potato Soup (see recipe page 78)
or any low-calorie soup up to 80 calories
50g (1¾oz) bread roll
'Twinpot' yogurt or similar diet yogurt with
fruit addition

— **OR** —

2 small low-fat sausages, grilled
175g (6oz) potato mashed with milk
from allowance
100g (3½oz) cabbage
1 satsuma

500 CALORIES — MAIN MEALS

Any ready meal or vegetarian ready meal up to
400 calories
200g (7oz) vegetables from low-calorie list
1 diet yogurt or 1 diet fromage frais
150g (5oz) piece of fresh fruit

— **OR** —

Stir-fried Thai Beef with noodles or rice
(see recipe page 90)
Green salad

— **OR** —

Meal Out or Takeaway Choice
1 small cheese and tomato pizza with vegetable
topping
Selection from salad bar
Note: No Extras calories with this choice

— **OR** —

1 Doner Kebab
Note: No Extras calories with this choice

300 CALORIES — EXTRAS

Anything up to 300 calories. All or part of this
allowance may be saved for another day.

Slimming tip: Making soup

Home-made soups are highly nutritious and economical to make. They taste better than canned ready-made ones, and you can control their calorie content. You will find some very low-calorie soup recipes on page 76. You can make soup in bulk when vegetables are cheap and plentiful, and then freeze it in individual portions until needed. This way you always have a supply handy when hunger pangs strike.

Soups are perfect for light meals and snacks when you are dieting. They are very filling and warming and can be made with almost any combination of vegetables. To make them more substantial, you can add some grated cheese, pasta shapes or beans but remember to count those extra calories. They soon add up!

DAY 7

250 CALORIES — MILK AND FAT ALLOWANCE

550ml (1 pint) skimmed milk
3 teaspoons low-fat spread or 1 teaspoon oil

— OR —

500ml (18 fl oz) semi-skimmed milk
2 teaspoons very low-fat spread
or ½ teaspoon oil

300 CALORIES — BREAKFASTS

60g (2oz) lean trimmed back bacon, grilled
1 size 4 egg, dry-fried or poached
Grilled tomatoes
30g (1oz) slice bread or toast
2 teaspoons low-sugar jam or 1 teaspoon honey

— OR —

Vegetarians may replace the bacon with 1
Potato Waffle, grilled or 30g (1oz) slice toast

300 CALORIES — LIGHT MEALS

Grecian-style Baked Fish (see recipe page 78)
Green salad
150g (5oz) new potatoes

— OR —

175g (6oz) potato, jacket baked or microwaved
150g (5oz) reduced-sugar and salt baked beans
Green salad
1 orange

500 CALORIES — MAIN MEALS

85g (3oz) lean roast meat
3 tablespoons thin low-fat gravy
1 small frozen Yorkshire pudding
or 1 tablespoon stuffing or apple sauce
175g (6oz) potato, dry roast or jacket baked
75g (2½oz) Brussels sprouts or broccoli
75g (2½oz) carrots
1 meringue nest topped with 2 tablespoons diet
yogurt, garnished with fruit

— OR —

Cheesey Vegetable Bake (see recipe page 43)
100g (3½oz) peas
200g (7oz) baked apple stuffed with
15g (½oz) raisins or 2 dates
2 tablespoons Greek yogurt
or 30g (1oz) ice cream

— OR —

Italian Stuffed Chicken (see recipe page 92)
100g (3½oz) canned fruit in juice
1 serving sugar-free jelly

300 CALORIES — EXTRAS

Anything up to 300 calories. All or part of this
allowance may be saved for another day.

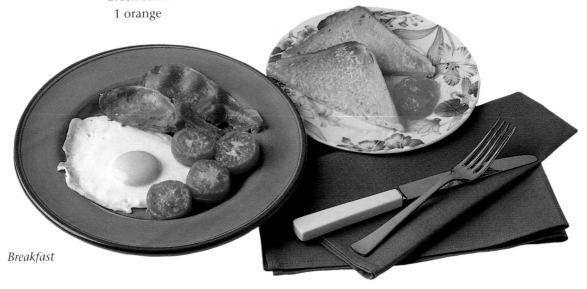

Breakfast

HIDDEN CALORIES

We eat many foods without thinking about the hidden calories that may be lurking within them. Look at the foods shown here – you may be surprised by the high calorie counts.

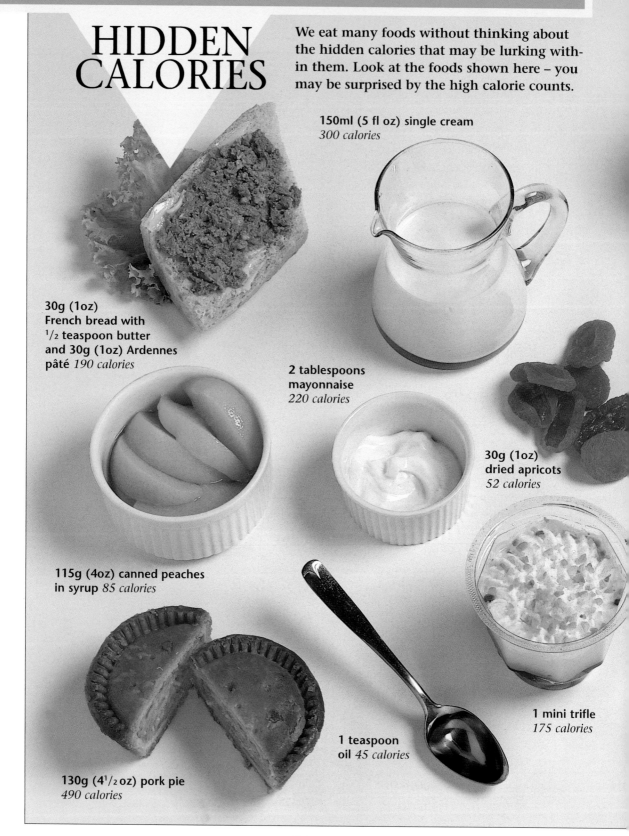

150ml (5 fl oz) single cream
300 calories

30g (1oz) French bread with ¹/₂ **teaspoon butter and 30g (1oz) Ardennes pâté** *190 calories*

2 tablespoons mayonnaise
220 calories

30g (1oz) dried apricots
52 calories

115g (4oz) canned peaches in syrup *85 calories*

1 mini trifle
175 calories

1 teaspoon oil *45 calories*

130g (4¹/₂oz) pork pie
490 calories

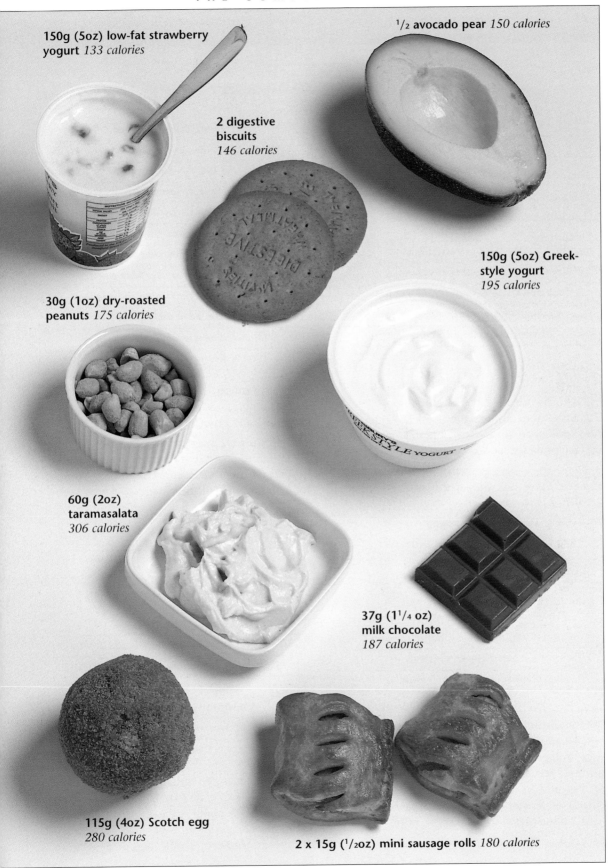

150g (5oz) low-fat strawberry yogurt *133 calories*

¹/₂ avocado pear *150 calories*

2 digestive biscuits *146 calories*

30g (1oz) dry-roasted peanuts *175 calories*

150g (5oz) Greek-style yogurt *195 calories*

60g (2oz) taramasalata *306 calories*

37g (1¹/₄ oz) milk chocolate *187 calories*

115g (4oz) Scotch egg *280 calories*

2 x 15g (¹/₂oz) mini sausage rolls *180 calories*

SPICY VEGETABLE SOUP

1 small onion, finely chopped
2 teaspoons oil
1 teaspoon ground cumin
1 teaspoon curry powder
1 teaspoon turmeric
225g (8oz) parsnips, diced
225g (8oz) carrots, diced
1 litre (1³/₄ pints) chicken or vegetable stock
salt and freshly ground black pepper
4 tablespoons low-fat natural yogurt
2 tablespoons chopped coriander

1 Sauté the onion in the oil until softened. Stir in the spices and cook for 2-3 minutes, stirring. Add the parsnips and carrots and stir well.

2 Add the stock and bring to the boil. Reduce the heat and simmer for about 20 minutes, or until the vegetables are tender. Season with salt and pepper.

3 Blend in a food processor or blender until smooth. Serve hot with a spoonful of yogurt, garnished with coriander.

Serves 4   *160 calories per serving*

———————— ◆◆◆ ————————

MINTY CUCUMBER SOUP

1 large cucumber, peeled and chopped
850ml (1¹/₂ pints) low-fat natural yogurt
1-2 garlic cloves, crushed
2 tablespoons chopped mint
salt and pepper

Put the cucumber in a colander and sprinkle with salt. Set aside for 1 hour, rinse under running cold water and press down to extract as much liquid as possible. Mix the yogurt with the garlic and half of the mint in a bowl, and stir in the drained cucumber. Season to taste and refrigerate for at least 2 hours. Serve sprinkled with mint.

Serves 4   *125 calories per serving*

MIXED VEGETABLE SOUP

1 onion, finely chopped
1 garlic clove, crushed (optional)
1 large carrot, diced
1 leek, shredded
2 celery sticks, chopped
1 red pepper, chopped
1 green pepper, chopped
850ml (1¹/₂ pints) vegetable stock
1 x 198g (7oz) can of chopped tomatoes
60g (2oz) shredded cabbage or lettuce
salt and freshly ground black pepper
2 tablespoons chopped fresh herbs

1 Put the onion, garlic (if using), carrot, leek, celery, peppers, stock and tomatoes in a large saucepan, and bring to the boil.

2 Lower the heat to a simmer, and cook gently for 20-25 minutes, until the vegetables are tender. Add the cabbage or lettuce and seasoning. Simmer for 5-10 minutes, and serve sprinkled with herbs.

Serves 4   *45 calories per serving*

———————— ◆◆◆ ————————

PINEAPPLE FRUIT SALAD

2 small pineapples
175g (6oz) strawberries, hulled and halved
115g (4oz) raspberries, thawed if frozen
115g (4oz) seedless grapes
1 kiwi fruit, peeled and diced
4 tablespoons orange juice
artificial sweetener, to taste (optional)

1 Cut the pineapples in half and cut around the sides with a sharp knife to remove the inner flesh, leaving a shell about 1.25cm (¹/₂ inch) thick. Scoop out the inside of each half, cut out and discard the hard central core, and dice the flesh.

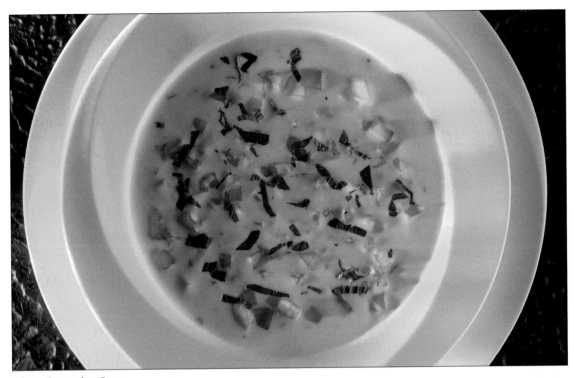

Minty Cucumber Soup

2 Put the diced pineapple, strawberries, raspberries, grapes and kiwi fruit in a bowl. Sprinkle with orange juice (sweetened if wished with artificial sweetener), and chill in the refrigerator for 1 hour.

3 Divide the fruit between the pineapple shells and serve immediately.

Serves 4   *105 calories per serving*

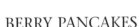

BERRY PANCAKES

For the pancakes:

115g (4oz) plain flour

pinch of salt

1 egg (size 1)

275ml (¹/₂ pint) skimmed milk

1 teaspoon oil for frying

FOR THE FILLING:

225g (8oz) very low-fat fromage frais

225g (8oz) strawberries, hulled and sliced, or raspberries or other berries

artificial sweetener, to taste

1 Make the pancakes: beat the flour, salt and egg together in a large bowl, and then gradually whisk in the milk. Alternatively, blend in a food processor or blender until smooth. Leave to stand for 30 minutes.

2 Heat a little of the oil in a small frying pan and, when it sizzles, pour in sufficient batter to cover the base thinly and evenly, tilting the pan. When the under-side is set and golden, flip the pancake over and cook the other side. Repeat with the remaining batter to make 8 small pancakes.

3 Mix together the fromage frais and berries, adding artificial sweetener to taste. Divide between the warm pancakes, and roll up or fold over to make cornets. Serve warm.

Serves 4   *200 calories per serving*

LEEK AND POTATO SOUP

2 medium leeks, washed, trimmed and chopped
1 small onion, chopped
175g (6oz) potato, peeled and diced
425ml ($^3/_4$ pint) chicken stock
275ml ($^1/_2$ pint) skimmed milk
salt and freshly ground black pepper
2 tablespoons chopped parsley or chives

1 Put the leeks, onion and potato in a large saucepan with the chicken stock. Bring to the boil, then reduce the heat and simmer gently for 20 minutes, until the vegetables are tender.

2 Add the skimmed milk, and then blend in a food processor or blender until smooth. Season to taste, and serve either hot or chilled, sprinkled with parsley or chives.

Serves 4   *80 calories per serving*

———— ◆◆◆ ————

GRECIAN-STYLE BAKED FISH

4 x 115g (4oz) cod steaks
2 tablespoons lemon juice
1 tablespoon olive oil
1 small onion, chopped
1 small bulb fennel, sliced (optional)
2 garlic cloves, crushed
2 teaspoons tomato paste
450g (1lb) tomatoes, skinned and chopped (or canned)
1 teaspoon chopped thyme
small sprig of rosemary
4 tablespoons red wine or stock
salt and freshly ground black pepper
8 black olives, to garnish (optional)

1 Wash the cod steaks, sprinkle with lemon juice and set aside.

2 Heat the oil and gently sauté the onion, fennel (if using) and garlic until softened and golden. Add the tomato paste, tomatoes, herbs and wine or stock. Season with salt and pepper, and simmer for 5 minutes.

3 Put the cod steaks in an ovenproof dish and pour the tomato sauce over the top. Bake in a preheated oven at 180°C/350°F/Gas Mark 4 for 20 minutes. Serve immediately, garnished if wished with black olives.

Serves 4   *170 calories per serving*

———— ◆◆◆ ————

ORANGE CHOCOLATE POTS

2 eggs (size 3)
2 tablespoons cocoa powder
425ml ($^3/_4$ pint) skimmed milk
2 tablespoons orange liqueur
artificial sweetener, to taste
60ml (2 fl oz) whipping cream
4 maraschino cherries or grated orange zest, to decorate

1 Whisk the eggs and cocoa powder together in a bowl until thoroughly blended. Heat the milk to boiling point, and then gradually whisk into the egg mixture.

2 Set the bowl over a saucepan of simmering water and cook, stirring constantly, until the mixture thickens. Stir in the orange liqueur and artificial sweetener to taste.

3 Pour the mixture into 4 ovenproof ramekin dishes and stand in a roasting pan with hot water half-way up the sides of the dishes. Cover with lightly greased foil, and bake in a preheated oven at 170°C/325°F/Gas Mark 3 for 25 minutes, or until set.

4 Remove from the oven, cool and chill. Whip the cream and use to decorate the chocolate pots. Decorate with cherries or grated orange zest.

Serves 4   *165 calories per serving*

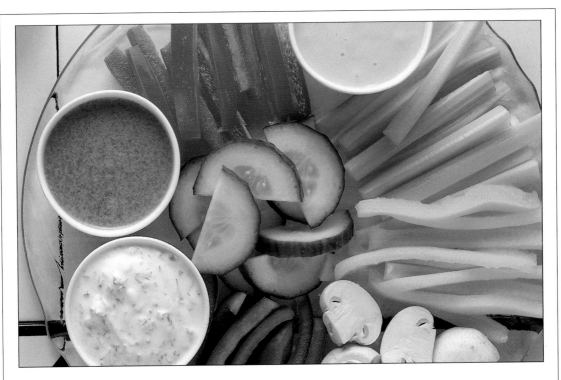

CRUDITES WITH DIPS

For the crudités

button mushrooms, halved

yellow, green and red peppers,
seeded and thinly sliced

cucumber, cut into chunks

celery, cut into sticks

Italian anchovy dip

5g (1¹/₂oz) can anchovy fillets, drained

1 garlic clove

1 tablespoon olive oil

1 tablespoon tomato paste

3 tablespoons low-calorie mayonnaise

Put all the ingredients in a blender or food processor and blend until smooth.

Serves 4   *95 calories per serving*

Garlic dip

100ml (3¹/₂ fl oz) very low-fat fromage frais

100ml (3¹/₂ fl oz) low-calorie mayonnaise

squeeze of lemon juice

2-3 garlic cloves, crushed

Mix all the ingredients together in a bowl until thoroughly blended.

Serves 4   *80 calories per serving*

Cheese, chive and herb dip

175g (6oz) low-fat soft cheese

2 tablespoons low-fat natural yogurt

4 tablespoons chopped fresh herbs

salt and freshly ground black pepper

Mix all the ingredients together in a bowl, seasoning to taste.

Serves 4   *80 calories per serving*

QUORN SPAGHETTI BOLOGNESE

225g (8oz) spaghetti

FOR THE SAUCE:
2 x 400g (14oz) cans of chopped tomatoes

1 onion, finely chopped

1 garlic clove, crushed

1 carrot, finely chopped

1 celery stick, finely chopped

4 tablespoons passata (sieved tomatoes)

a little vegetable stock

1 teaspoon chopped fresh thyme

225g (8oz) minced Quorn

salt and freshly ground black pepper

$^1/_2$ teaspoon sugar

1 Put all the ingredients for the sauce in a saucepan and simmer for 20 minutes, adding more stock if necessary.

2 Cook the spaghetti in plenty of boiling, lightly salted water until tender but still firm. Drain well and serve with the sauce.

Serves 4   *295 calories per serving*

—————— ◆ ◆ ◆ ——————

DEVILLED TURKEY AND MANGE TOUT SALAD

175g (6oz) mange tout, trimmed

350g (12oz) cooked turkey or chicken

1 red pepper, seeded and diced

1 yellow pepper, seeded and diced

30g (1oz) nuts, e.g. pine nuts, peanuts

1 kiwi fruit, peeled and sliced

FOR THE DRESSING:
1 tablespoon olive oil

1 tablespoon wine vinegar

1 tablespoon lemon juice

1 teaspoon Worcestershire sauce

$^1/_2$ teaspoon paprika

$^1/_2$ teaspoon mustard

pinch of ground cumin

salt and freshly ground black pepper

1 Cut the mange tout in half. Cover with boiling water. and leave to stand for 2 minutes. Drain and rinse.

2 Put the mange tout in a serving bowl with the turkey or chicken, peppers and nuts.

3 Make the dressing and toss the salad. Serve garnished with sliced kiwi fruit.

Serves 4   *245 calories per serving*

—————— ◆ ◆ ◆ ——————

MEDITERRANEAN FISH STEW

450g (1lb) mixed fish, e.g. cod, haddock, monkfish, squid

225g (8oz) shellfish, e.g. prawns, fresh or canned mussels

2 tablespoons oil

1 onion, chopped

1 fennel bulb, sliced (optional)

2 garlic cloves, crushed

2 medium potatoes, peeled and diced

3 tomatoes, skinned and chopped

few strips of orange zest

1.1 litre (2 pints) fish stock

salt and freshly ground black pepper

1 Clean and prepare the fish, removing any skin and bones and cutting into chunks. Shell the prawns and scrub the mussels (if using fresh).

2 Heat the oil in a large saucepan and sauté the onion, fennel (if using) and garlic until soft. Add the fish, potatoes, tomatoes, orange zest, stock and seasoning. Bring to the boil, and then simmer for 15 minutes. Add the shellfish and cook for 5 minutes.

Serves 4   *285 calories per serving*

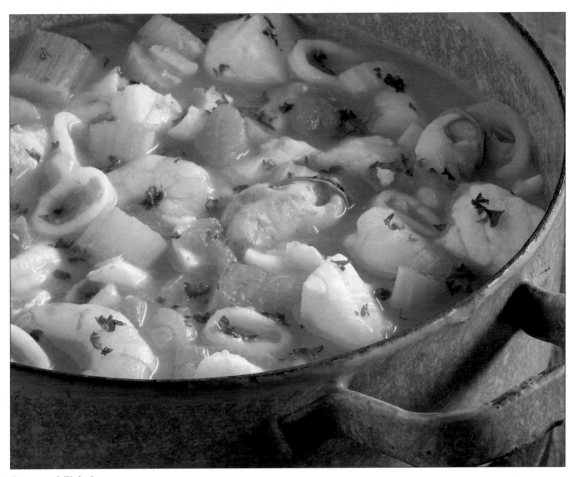

Provençal Fish Soup

PROVENCAL FISH SOUP

1 onion, chopped

1 celery stick, chopped

1 garlic clove, crushed

1 tablespoon olive oil

450g (1lb) white fish of your choice, e.g. cod, haddock, monkfish, cubed

450g (1lb) tomatoes, skinned and chopped (or use canned)

¹/₂ teaspoon sugar

1 teaspoon dried mixed herbs, preferably Herbes de Provence

1 small packet of powdered saffron

salt and freshly ground black pepper

550ml (1 pint) fish stock

225g (8oz) fresh or frozen seafood, e.g. prawns, squid

2 tablespoons chopped parsley

1 Sauté the onion, celery and garlic in the olive oil until soft and golden – do not brown. Add the fish, tomatoes, sugar, herbs, saffron, seasoning and stock, and bring to the boil. Cover the pan and simmer for 5 minutes.

2 Add the seafood, return to the boil, and then reduce the heat and simmer for a further 2 minutes. Serve the soup immediately sprinkled with parsley.

Serves 4 *225 calories per serving*

CHINESE SALAD

$^1/_2$ head Chinese leaves

85g (3oz) spinach, shredded

115g (4oz) cooked baby sweetcorn

5cm (2-inch) piece of cucumber, cut into sticks

5 spring onions, shredded

8 radishes, sliced

60g (2oz) bean sprouts

115g (4oz) cooked chicken, shredded

1 teaspoon sesame seeds

FOR THE DRESSING:

1 tablespoon sunflower oil

2 tablespoons light soy sauce

pinch of chilli powder

1 Shred the Chinese leaves and put them in a bowl with the salad vegetables and chicken.

2 Make the dressing and toss with the salad. Serve sprinkled with sesame seeds.

Serves 2   *250 calories per serving*

CURRIED VEGETABLES

1 onion, chopped

2 garlic cloves, crushed

1 tablespoon oil

2 teaspoons curry powder

2 teaspoons ground coriander

$^1/_2$ teaspoon turmeric

450g (1lb) prepared vegetables, e.g. diced potato, diced carrot, cauliflower florets, thin green beans

450g (1lb) tomatoes, skinned and chopped (or use canned)

115g (4oz) mushrooms, quartered

150ml ($^1/_4$ pint) vegetable stock

115g (4oz) frozen peas

150ml ($^1/_4$ pint) low-fat natural yogurt

60g (2oz) cucumber, diced

2 spring onions, thinly sliced

1 fresh green chilli, seeded and chopped (optional)

coriander leaves, to garnish

Chinese Salad

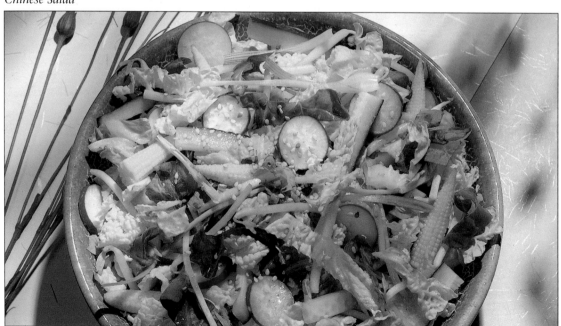

175g (6oz) brown rice (raw weight), boiled

1 Sauté the onion and garlic in the oil until tender and golden. Add the spices and cook, stirring, for 2 minutes.

2 Add the prepared vegetables, tomatoes, mushrooms, stock and peas. Cover the pan and simmer gently for 20-25 minutes, until the vegetables are cooked and tender.

3 Meanwhile, mix the yogurt with the cucumber, spring onions and chilli. Serve with the curried vegetables, sprinkled with coriander, with rice.

Serves 4   *300 calories per serving*

— ◆◆◆ —

STUFFED COURGETTES

225g (8oz) long-grain brown rice

6 spring onions, chopped

115g (4oz) mushrooms, chopped

1 garlic clove, crushed

700ml (1¼ pints) vegetable stock

2 tomatoes, skinned and chopped

1 tablespoon chopped herbs,
e.g. oregano, basil, parsley

salt and freshly ground black pepper

4 x 225g (8oz) courgettes

15g (½oz) grated Cheddar cheese

1 Put the rice, spring onions, mushrooms and garlic in a saucepan with the vegetable stock and bring to the boil. Reduce the heat , cover the pan and simmer gently for about 45 minutes. The rice should be cooked and all the liquid absorbed. Stir in the tomatoes and chopped herbs, and season to taste.

2 Cook the courgettes in boiling water for 4-5 minutes. Remove and drain. Cut them in half lengthways and scoop out and discard the seeds. Pile the rice into the courgette shells, and sprinkle with cheese. Pop under a preheated hot grill until the cheese is golden and bubbling.

Serves 4   *260 calories per serving*

LAMB CURRY

1 onion, sliced

2 garlic cloves, crushed

3 dried red chilli peppers

1 tablespoon ground coriander

2 teaspoons ground cumin

1 teaspoon ground cinnamon

200ml (7 fl oz) water

150g (5oz) low-fat natural yogurt

450g (1lb) lean lamb, cubed

orange wedges, to garnish

FOR THE RICE:

115g (4oz) basmati rice

700ml (1¼ pints) boiling water

2 celery sticks, finely chopped

salt and freshly ground black pepper

1 Put the onion, garlic, spices, water, yogurt and lamb in a saucepan, and bring to the boil. Cover the pan and simmer gently for 1¼ hours. Remove the lid and boil rapidly for 5-10 minutes to reduce the liquid. Discard the chilli peppers.

2 Rinse the rice in a sieve under running cold water. Put the rice in a large saucepan with the boiling water and return to the boil. Cook, uncovered, for 12-14 minutes. Drain and rinse with boiling water, and stir in the celery. Season to taste.

3 Serve the lamb curry with the rice, garnished with orange wedges.

Serves 4   *285 calories per serving*

Slimming tip

If you make your own curries, you can control the calories better than if you eat in an Indian restaurant or buy a take-away.

TORTELLONI PRIMAVERA

300g (10oz) fresh tortelloni

85g (3oz) grated Parmesan cheese

FOR THE SAUCE:

450g (1lb) fresh or frozen broccoli

4 tablespoons skimmed milk

salt and freshly ground black pepper

1 Make the sauce: cook the broccoli in boiling, lightly salted water until tender. If using frozen broccoli, follow the instructions on the packet. Drain well and add the milk and seasoning.

2 Cook the tortelloni in boiling, lightly salted water until just tender but still firm. Drain well and mix into the broccoli sauce. Toss together with some of the Parmesan, and serve sprinkled with the remaining Parmesan.

Serves 4   *300 calories per serving*

Variation: *You can vary the green vegetables in this recipe by substituting mange tout, asparagus or thin green beans (or a mixture of all three) for the broccoli.*

◆◆◆

ITALIAN HUNTER'S CHICKEN

1 tablespoon olive oil

4 x 250g (9oz) chicken portions, skin removed

1 red onion, roughly chopped

1 garlic clove, crushed

450g (1lb) tomatoes, skinned and chopped

115g (4oz) button mushrooms, sliced

2 bay leaves

1 sprig of rosemary

150ml (^{1}/$_4$ pint) dry white wine

275ml (^{1}/$_2$ pint) chicken stock

salt and freshly ground black pepper

1 Heat the oil in a large frying pan and sauté the chicken, turning occasionally, until golden on all sides. Remove from the pan and keep warm.

2 Add the red onion, garlic, tomatoes and mushrooms, and cook gently until softened. Add the bay leaves, rosemary, wine and stock, and return the chicken to the pan. Simmer for about 45 minutes, or until the chicken is cooked and tender and the sauce reduced. Season with salt and pepper and serve.

Serves 4   *300 calories per serving*

◆◆◆

SAUSAGE HOTPOT

225g (8oz) lean pork fillet, cubed

1 onion, chopped

1 garlic clove, crushed

1 large carrot, thickly sliced

1 tablespoon oil

400g (14oz) canned chopped tomatoes

275ml (^{1}/$_2$ pint) beef stock

salt and freshly ground black pepper

2 large low-fat pork sausages, thickly sliced

225g (8oz) canned white haricot beans, drained

60g (2oz) dried breadcrumbs

1 Cook the pork in its own fat in a non-stick pan until lightly browned all over. Drain off any fat.

2 Sauté the onion, garlic and carrot in the oil until softened. Add the tomatoes, beef stock and seasoning and bring to the boil. Reduce the heat and add the pork and sausages. Simmer gently for 20 minutes until cooked and reduced.

3 Stir in the beans and transfer to an ovenproof dish. Sprinkle with breadcrumbs and bake in a preheated oven at 180°C/350°F/Gas Mark 4 for 15-20 minutes, until crisp and golden brown.

Serves 4   *260 calories per serving*

CHEESE AND SPINACH SALAD

225g (8oz) low-fat soft cheese

60g (2oz) walnuts, chopped

225g (8oz) spinach leaves, washed and trimmed

3 sticks celery, sliced

5cm (2-inch) piece of cucumber, diced

1 dessert apple, cored and diced

1 tablespoon lemon juice

1 tablespoon white wine vinegar

1 tablespoon olive oil

salt and freshly ground black pepper

1 Make the cheese balls: take teaspoonfuls of cheese and mould into balls. Roll them in the chopped nuts and chill until required.

2 Put the spinach, celery and cucumber in a bowl. Toss the apple in the lemon juice, drain and add to the spinach. Mix the vinegar and oil with the remaining lemon juice. Season and gently toss the salad in this dressing. Add the cheese balls and serve.

Serves 4   *260 calories per serving*

Cheese and Spinach Salad

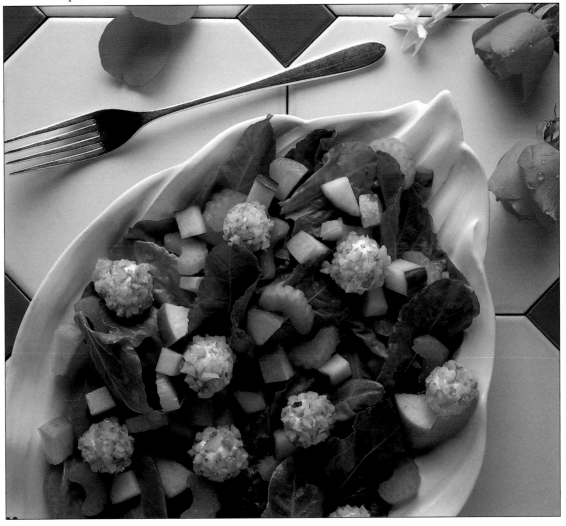

BUTTER BEAN BAKE

15g (¹/₂oz) soft margarine

1 small onion, finely chopped

115g (4oz) button mushrooms, halved

30g (1oz) plain flour

275ml (¹/₂ pint) skimmed milk

pinch of ground nutmeg

salt and freshly ground black pepper

450g (1lb) cooked butter beans (rinsed and drained if canned)

2 tomatoes, sliced

30g (1oz) grated half-fat Cheddar cheese

1 Melt the margarine in a saucepan, and sauté the onion and mushrooms until tender. Stir in the plain flour and cook gently over low heat for 1-2 minutes.

2 Gradually add the milk, stirring well, and bring to the boil. Reduce the heat and add the nutmeg and seasoning to taste. Add the butter beans.

3 Pour half the mixture into a heatproof dish, cover with a layer of tomato, and top with the remaining sauce. Sprinkle with cheese and place under a hot grill until golden and bubbling.

Serves 2   *395 calories per serving*

———————— ◆◆◆ ————————

SWEET AND SOUR PORK

375g (12oz) lean pork fillet, cubed

2 teaspoons oil

1 onion , thinly sliced

1 red pepper, seeded and cut into chunks

1 carrot, thinly sliced

225ml (8 fl oz) chicken or vegetable stock

60g (2oz) mange tout

2 tomatoes, skinned and cut into quarters

2 pineapple rings (canned in natural juice), cut into chunks

2 tablespoons soy sauce

2 tablespoons unsweetened pineapple juice

1 tablespoon vinegar

2 teaspoons brown sugar

1 tablespoon cornflour

175g (6oz) rice (raw weight), boiled

1 Cook the pork quickly in the oil, turning to brown the cubes all over. Add the onion, pepper and carrot, and stir-fry for 2 minutes. Pour in the stock, and simmer over low heat for 15-20 minutes, until the pork is cooked.

2 Add the mange tout, tomatoes and pineapple and cook for a further 5 minutes. Mix the soy sauce, pineapple juice, vinegar, brown sugar and cornflour together, and then stir into the pork mixture. Continue stirring over low heat until the sauce thickens. Serve with boiled rice.

Serves 4   *345 calories per serving*

———————— ◆◆◆ ————————

PASTA WITH TOMATO SAUCE

1 tablespoon olive oil

1 onion, finely chopped

2 garlic cloves, crushed

450g (1lb) tomatoes, skinned and chopped

2 tablespoons tomato paste

3-4 tablespoons white or red wine

6 olives, stoned and quartered (optional)

a few basil leaves, shredded (or 1 teaspoon dried basil)

salt and freshly ground black pepper

275g (10oz) tagliatelle

4 tablespoons grated Parmesan cheese

a few basil leaves, to garnish

1 Heat the oil and sauté the onion and garlic until softened. Add the tomatoes, tomato paste and wine, and cook gently over low heat for about 15

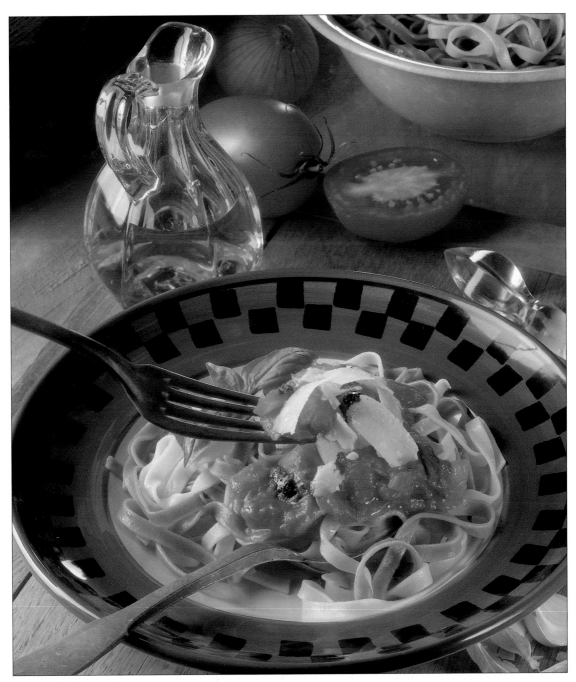

Pasta with Tomato Sauce

minutes, until the sauce is thick and reduced. Add the olives and basil, and season to taste.

2 Meanwhile, cook the tagliatelle in plenty of lightly salted boiling water until just tender but still firm. Drain well and serve with the tomato sauce. Sprinkle with Parmesan cheese and garnish with basil.

Serves 4   *360 calories per serving*

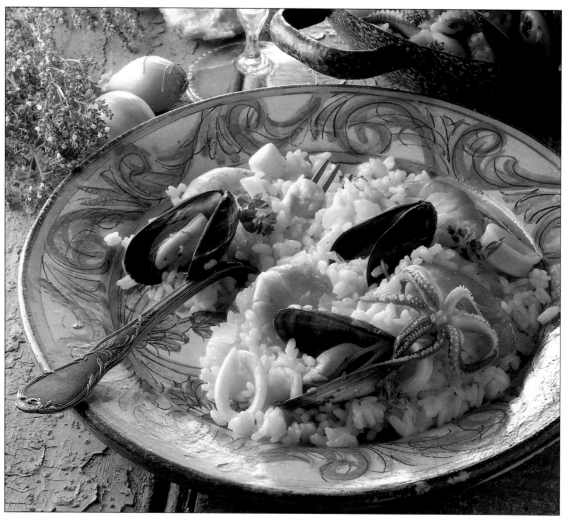

Seafood Risotto

SEAFOOD RISOTTO

450g (1lb) fresh mussels in their shells

1 tablespoon olive oil

1 onion, chopped

2 garlic cloves, crushed

225g (8oz) Arborio risotto rice

850ml (1¹/₂ pints) fish stock

3 tablespoons dry white wine

225g (8oz) unpeeled cooked prawns, heads removed

225g (8oz) prepared squid, sliced

salt and freshly ground black pepper

sprigs of oregano, to garnish

1 Scrub the mussels and discard any with cracked shells. Cook in a covered pan of boiling water, shaking occasionally, until they open. Strain, reserving the cooking liquid, and discard any mussels that fail to open.

2 Heat the olive oil in a large deep frying pan and sauté the onion and garlic until softened. Stir in the rice and cook over low heat for 1 minute. Pour in a little of the fish stock, reserved mussel liquid and wine, stirring well. Bring to

the boil, then reduce the heat to a simmer and cook gently until the rice is tender and plump. Add more fish stock when necessary and stir occasionally to prevent the rice sticking.

3 After 15 minutes, add the prawns and squid. When the rice is cooked and all the liquid absorbed, season to taste and stir in the mussels in their shells. Heat through gently and serve garnished with sprigs of oregano.

Serves 4   *370 calories per serving*

———— ◆◆ ◆ ————

VEGETABLE CREPES

115g (4oz) plain flour, sifted
pinch of salt
1 egg, beaten
300ml (¹/₂ pint) skimmed milk
2 teaspoons oil
60g (2oz) grated half-fat Cheddar cheese

FOR THE FILLING:

175g (6oz) finely chopped onion
115g (4oz) mushrooms, thinly sliced
1 garlic clove, crushed
2 teaspoons oil
1 x 198g (7oz) can of chopped tomatoes
1 x 400g (14oz) can of kidney beans, rinsed and drained
salt and pepper
2 tablespoons chopped parsley

1 Make the crêpes: put the flour and salt in a mixing bowl and beat in the egg and milk to make a thick, smooth batter. Heat a little of the oil in a frying pan and pour in a little batter. Swirl it around, tilting the pan to cover the base. When it is set underneath, flip the crêpe over and cook the other side. Remove and keep warm while you make the remaining crêpes in the same way.

2 Make the filling: sauté the onion, mushrooms and garlic in the oil until soft. Add the tomatoes

and bring to the boil. Simmer gently for 10-15 minutes, until thickened and reduced. Stir in the kidney beans and season to taste. Add the parsley.

3 Fill the crêpes with the sauce and roll up. Sprinkle with cheese and flash under a hot grill until melted and golden.

Serves 4   *320 calories per serving*

———— ◆◆ ◆ ————

MEDITERRANEAN VEGETABLE PASTA

175g (6oz) chopped onion
1 garlic clove, crushed
225g (8oz) courgettes, cut into chunks
1 large aubergine, diced
1 large green pepper, seeded and diced
1 x 400g (14oz) can of chopped tomatoes
4 tablespoons passata (sieved tomatoes)
1 tablespoon chopped fresh basil or oregano
a little vegetable stock
225g (8oz) small florets of cauliflower
salt and freshly ground black pepper
300g (10oz) pasta shells (dry weight)
4 tablespoons grated Parmesan cheese

1 Put the onion, garlic, courgettes, aubergine, pepper and tomatoes into a large saucepan. Add the passata and herbs, cover the pan with a tight-fitting lid and simmer gently for about 30 minutes, or until the vegetables are cooked and tender. Stir occasionally and add a little stock if necessary to keep the vegetables moist.

2 Add the cauliflower, bring to the boil, and then simmer for 5 minutes. Season to taste.

3 Meanwhile, cook the pasta shells in boiling, lightly salted water until just tender but still firm. Drain well, and serve topped with the vegetable sauce sprinkled with Parmesan cheese.

Serves 4   *360 calories per serving*

CHICKEN WITH PEANUT SATAY SAUCE

450g (1lb) boneless chicken breasts, skinned
1 small onion, chopped
1 garlic clove, crushed
1 tablespoon light soy sauce
$^1/_2$ teaspoon each ground ginger and coriander
1 tablespoon oil
sliced cucumber and shredded spring onions, to garnish

FOR THE PEANUT SATAY SAUCE:

60g (2oz) unsalted roasted peanuts
1 tablespoon chunky peanut butter
1 garlic clove, crushed
1 tablespoon desiccated coconut
$^1/_2$ teaspoon hot chilli sauce
1 teaspoon sugar
115ml (4 fl oz) low-fat fromage frais
175g (6oz) brown rice (raw weight), boiled

1 Cut the chicken into cubes and put in a bowl. Mix together the onion, garlic, soy sauce, ginger, coriander and oil. Pour over the chicken and stir well. Cover and refrigerate for 2 hours.

2 Thread the chicken onto bamboo skewers and place under a hot grill or on a barbecue for 6-8 minutes, turning occasionally, until cooked and evenly brown.

3 Meanwhile, put all the ingredients for the peanut satay sauce in a blender or food processor and blend until smooth. Serve with the chicken kebabs, garnished with sliced cucumber and shredded spring onions. Serve with boiled rice.

Serves 4   *490 calories per serving*

CHILLI CON CARNE

450g (1lb) lean minced beef
2 teaspoons oil
1 onion, chopped
1 garlic clove, crushed
1 green pepper, seeded and chopped
1-2 fresh chillies, seeded and chopped
400g (14oz) canned chopped tomatoes
1 tablespoon tomato paste
150ml ($^1/_4$ pint) beef stock
425g (15oz) can red kidney beans, rinsed and drained
salt and pepper
1 tablespoon chopped coriander (optional)
175g (6oz) rice (raw weight), boiled

1 Cook the minced beef in its own fat in a non-stick pan until browned. Drain off the fat.

2 Heat the oil in a saucepan and sauté the onion, garlic and green pepper for about 5 minutes, until softened. Add the chilli and stir-fry for 1 minute.

3 Add the tomatoes, tomato paste and beef stock, and bring to the boil. Lower the heat and simmer for 30 minutes until thickened and reduced. Stir in the kidney beans and heat through gently. Season to taste. Serve garnished with coriander with the boiled rice.

Serves 4   *480 calories per serving*

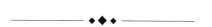

STIR-FRIED THAI BEEF

1 tablespoon oil
1 onion, thinly sliced
1 garlic clove, crushed
2.5cm (1-inch) fresh root ginger, chopped (optional)
450g (1lb) lean rump steak, sliced thinly
1 tablespoon soy sauce
1 red pepper, seeded and sliced

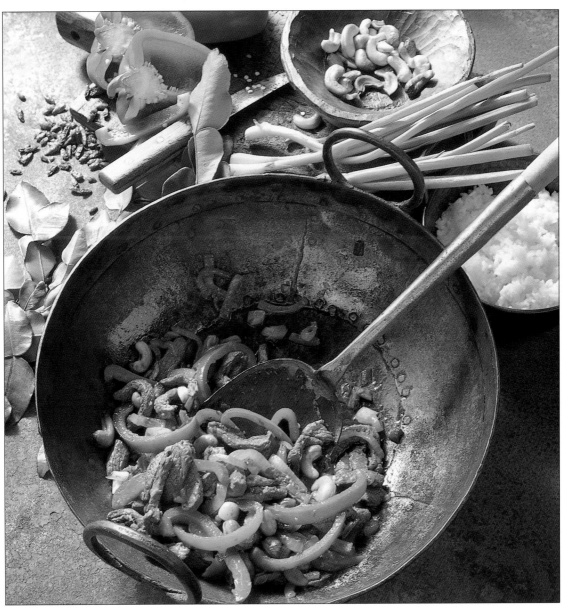

Stir-fried Thai Beef

1 green pepper, seeded and sliced

1 red chilli, seeded and chopped

4 spring onions, sliced diagonally

60g (2oz) cashews or unroasted peanuts

175g (6oz) Chinese noodles or rice
(raw weight), boiled

1 Heat the oil in a wok or frying pan and stir-fry the onion, garlic and ginger for 3 minutes. Add the strips of steak and stir-fry for 2 minutes.

2 Stir in the soy sauce and add the peppers, chilli and spring onions. Stir-fry for 2-3 minutes and then stir in the cashews or peanuts. Serve with boiled rice or noodles.

Serves 4 *490 calories per serving*

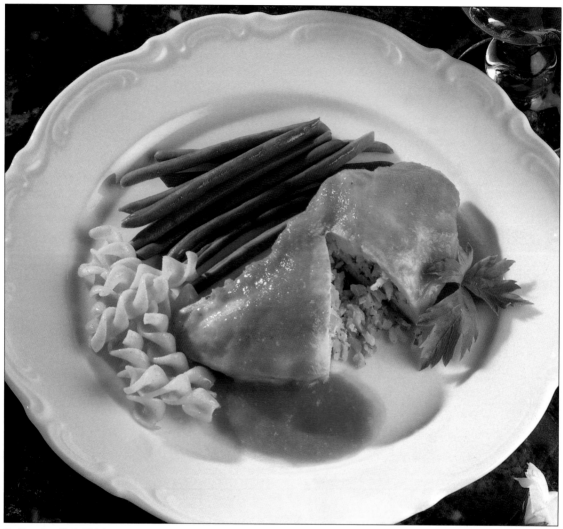

Italian Stuffed Chicken

ITALIAN STUFFED CHICKEN

4 boneless chicken breasts, skinned

30g (1oz) cooked lean ham, diced

60g (2oz) cooked rice

1 tablespoon chopped parsley

$^1/_2$ egg, beaten

salt and pepper

1 tablespoon low-fat spread

150ml ($^1/_4$ pint) chicken stock

3 tablespoons dry white wine

2 tablespoons tomato paste

225g (8oz) dried pasta shapes

1 Cut a slit in each chicken breast to make a pocket. Mix together the ham, rice, parsley and beaten egg, and season with salt and pepper. Fill the chicken 'pockets' with this mixture and secure with cocktail sticks.

2 Heat the fat in a non-stick frying pan and sauté the chicken breasts until golden on both sides.

Pour the stock and wine over the chicken and stir in the tomato paste. Bring to the boil, then cover and simmer for about 20 minutes, until the chicken is cooked and tender.

3 Remove the chicken and keep warm. Boil the pan juices to reduce and thicken them, and pour over the chicken.

4 Meanwhile, cook the pasta in plenty of lightly salted boiling water until tender but still firm. Drain well and serve with the chicken.

Serve 4   *425 calories per serving*

◆◆◆

SPAGHETTI BOLOGNESE

450g (1lb) very lean minced beef
1 small onion, chopped
2 carrots, diced
2 garlic cloves, crushed
2 teaspoons oil
450g (1lb) tomatoes, skinned and chopped (or use canned)
150ml ($^1/_4$ pint) passata (sieved tomatoes)
150ml ($^1/_4$ pint) beef stock
$^1/_2$ teaspoon dried oregano
salt and freshly ground black pepper
225g (8oz) spaghetti

1 Fry the minced beef in its own fat in a non-stick pan until browned, and then drain off all the fat. Set aside.

2 Sauté the onion, carrots and garlic in the oil until softened. Add the tomatoes, passata, beef stock and oregano and bring to the boil. Reduce the heat and stir in the minced beef. Simmer for 30 minutes until thickened and reduced. Season to taste. Stir occasionally to prevent the sauce sticking to the pan.

3 Cook the spaghetti in plenty of lightly salted boiling water until just tender but still firm. Drain well and serve with the Bolognese sauce.

Serves 4   *470 calories per serving*

VEGETABLE CHILLI

1 onion, chopped
2 garlic cloves, crushed
2 teaspoons oil
1 red pepper, seeded and chopped
1 green pepper, seeded and chopped
1 medium aubergine, cut into chunks
2 courgettes, sliced
2 fresh chillies, seeded and chopped
400g (14oz) canned chopped tomatoes
150ml (1/4 pint) vegetable stock
425g (15oz) can red kidney beans, rinsed and drained
salt and pepper
85g (3oz) grated half-fat cheese
1 tablespoon chopped coriander (optional)
225g (8oz) rice (raw weight), boiled

1 Sauté the onion and garlic in the oil until soft. Add the peppers, aubergine, courgettes and chillies, and cook for 3-4 minutes. Add the chilli and cook for 1 minute.

2 Add the tomatoes and stock, and bring to the boil. Simmer for 30 minutes until thickened and reduced. Stir in the kidney beans and heat through gently. Season to taste and serve the chilli sprinkled with cheese and coriander, with boiled rice.

Serves 4   *400 calories per serving*

Slimming tip

This Vegetable Chilli recipe is a good way of using up any vegetables that may be lurking at the back of the fridge. You can vary the vegetables by substituting carrots, fresh tomatoes, mushrooms, celery or any vegetables from the low-calorie list (see page 25).

CHEESES

Cheese is a delicious snack when you feel like nibbling something, but most varieties tend to be high in fat – and calories! Always weigh the portions of cheese that you cut; most of us find it hard to judge a 30g (1oz) slice and wildly over-estimate.

30g (1oz) Cheddar cheese
120 calories

30g (1oz) Stilton
120 calories

30g (1oz) full-fat soft cheese *130 calories*

20g (3/4oz) Boursin with herbs
81 calories

30g (1oz) Red Leicester
118 calories

30g (1oz) Gruyère
120 calories

30g (1oz) Double Gloucester
118 calories

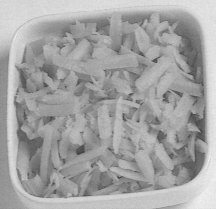

30g (1oz) Gorgonzola
105 calories

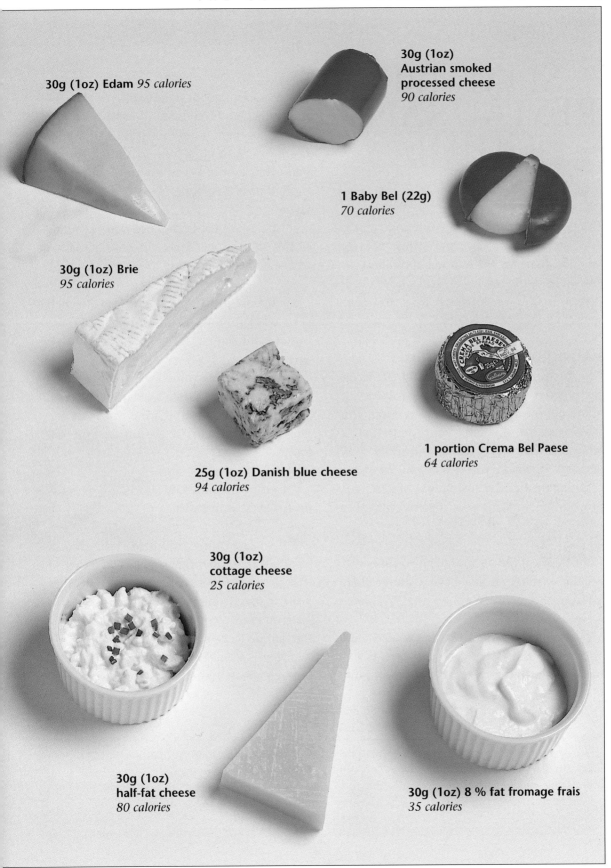

30g (1oz) Edam *95 calories*

**30g (1oz)
Austrian smoked
processed cheese**
90 calories

1 Baby Bel (22g)
70 calories

30g (1oz) Brie
95 calories

1 portion Crema Bel Paese
64 calories

25g (1oz) Danish blue cheese
94 calories

**30g (1oz)
cottage cheese**
25 calories

**30g (1oz)
half-fat cheese**
80 calories

30g (1oz) 8 % fat fromage frais
35 calories

SLIMMER RESTAURANT GUIDE

You need not ruin your diet and undo all the good work you have achieved just because you are going to eat out at a restaurant, or you've been invited to a friend's house. It is just a matter of learning how to make sensible low-calorie choices.

Eating out in restaurants

You can enjoy your meal without piling on the calories. If you are looking forward to going out for a special celebratory meal, you may wish to save up your daily Extras allowances for this occasion and really spoil yourself. However, you should still be aware of eating the healthy, low-fat way, and let this be your guide. Some good tips to remember when dining out are:

1 Cut down on the number of courses you eat: for example, if you have a starter, then give the dessert a miss.

2 Don't be tempted by the cheeseboard and opt for this rather than a dessert. It will be far higher in calories than some fresh fruit.

3 Be careful about your choice of starter – many are very high in fat. If possible, choose a clear vegetable soup or a salad, but ask for the dressing to be served separately so that you can use only a tiny amount – say, no to more than a teaspoon.

4 Opt for grilled, poached and steamed dishes if possible. Avoid fried and roasted foods, however tempting.

5 Choose plain dishes, and avoid rich calorie-laden sauces made with cream, flour, butter, wine or brandy.

6 Don't drink too much wine. Enjoy a glass with your meal and then have mineral water. Alternatively, water your wine down, as the French do, to make it go further and last longer.

7 Don't be tempted by chocolates or petits fours served with coffee.

8 If you are eating at a friend's house, don't be afraid to tell her that you are on a diet so that she can prepare some low-calorie dishes if she wishes. Don't be embarrassed about this – a true friend won't mind and will be only too willing to help and encourage you

Here is a quick at-a-glance guide to eating out in some of your favourite restaurants.

Party survival guide

- Eat before you go – don't arrive hungry.
- Sip diet drinks or low-alcohol wines or beers.
- Don't nibble high-calorie peanuts, crisps, sausage rolls, pastry canapes.

- Opt for low-calorie crudités and cottage cheese or fromage frais dips.
- Save some calories from your Extras allowance and use them carefully .

Italian restaurants

Mediterranean food is currently very fashionable and is extremely healthy with its emphasis on fresh vegetables, fruit, fish, grains, pulses, meat and poultry. However, like the Greeks, the Italians are extremely partial to olive oil and you must be on your guard when reading the menu. Surprisingly, pasta is the slimmer's friend, so long as it is tossed with a low-calorie tomato-based sauce rather than a rich creamy one.

 BEWARE OF:

✖ Risotto, which is usually cooked with oil, butter and cheese

✖ Salami and other fatty meats and sausages

✖ Cheeses, especially high-fat Parmesan which is grated and sprinkled over many soups, pasta and savoury dishes

✖ Deep-fried vegetables

✖ Creamy and buttery sauces for pasta

✖ Oily dressings on salads

✖ Lasagne and cannelloni, which are cloaked in creamy cheese sauces

✖ Fried meat, escalopes and fish

✖ Italian ice cream

✖ Tiramisu, zuppa inglese and other creamy Italian desserts

 CHOOSE:

✔ Pasta as a main course (not as a starter) with a tomato sauce

✔ Vegetable soups, e.g. Minestrone

✔ Pizza, if the crust is thin and crisp (not deep pan)

✔ Grilled fish, poultry and meat

✔ Salads, with dressing served separately

✔ Fresh fruit

French restaurants

Unfortunately, many classic French dishes tend to be high in calories, as the French are very liberal with cream, butter and wine. However, although there are several dishes that are out-of-bounds to slimmers, you can still enjoy your meal.

 BEWARE OF:

✖ Creamy soups

✖ Fritters, tartlets, quiches and pastries, which are often filled with sweet or savoury creamy mixtures

✖ Mousses and soufflés

✖ Pâtés and foie gras

✖ Oily hollandaise and mayonnaise sauces

✖ Fish fried in butter, e.g. meunière

✖ Meat, poultry and fish in creamy sauces, e.g. béchamel, mornay, velouté

✖ Dishes with full-fat cheese, e.g. gratins

✖ Ice creams

✖ Crème brulée, crème caramel and other sweet, creamy custards

 CHOOSE:

✔ Mussels, e.g. moules marinière

✔ Consommé and clear soups

✔ Grilled fish, meat and poultry

✔ Salads, but with dressing served separately

✔ Fresh fruit desserts and sorbets

Greek restaurants

Greek food has a reputation for being very healthy because it utilizes few dairy products, but it is also loaded with calories as most Greek cooks tend to be over-zealous with olive oil. You must take particular care when choosing a first course, as most starters are very oily or fried.

 BEWARE OF:

✖ Dips, e.g. taramasalata, hummus and aubergine purée – all are high in olive oil

✖ Tahini

✖ Sausages and sheftalia

✖ Spanakopitta (pastries filled with cheese)

✖ Fried squid and cheese, e.g. Haloumi

✖ Moussaka, often topped with a creamy sauce

✖ Dolmades, which are cooked in oil

✖ Tzatziki – this is made with Greek yogurt which is not as low in fat as other types, e.g. low-fat and diet yogurts

✖ Honey-laden desserts

✖ Sweetened Greek coffee

 CHOOSE:

✔ Avgolemono (chicken, egg and lemon soup)

✔ Grilled fish, chicken, lamb or pork

✔ Grilled kebabs

✔ Rice dishes

✔ Salads, with dressing served separately

✔ Pitta bread

✔ Unsweetened Greek coffee

Indian restaurants

You will probably be surprised to learn that many Indian dishes are out-of-bounds to slimmers. Even dishes made with yogurt can be relatively high in fat.

 BEWARE OF:

✖ Kormas and other dishes made with cream or cream cheese

✖ Samosas

✖ Onion bhajis

✖ Biriyanis which usually contain nuts and yogurt

✖ Deep-fried puri and poppadums

✖ Fried paratha

✖ Dishes made with coconut milk

✖ Fruit desserts in syrup

✖ Sherbets made with sugar

 CHOOSE:

✔ Dhal and lentil dishes

✔ Rice pullao

✔ Vegetable curries

✔ Vindaloos

✔ Kebabs

✔ Tandoori chicken

✔ Salads

Chinese restaurants

It is best to choose steamed and stir-fried dishes, and to pass on the deep-fried ones such as spring rolls.

BEWARE OF:

✖ Fried rice, egg-fried rice

✖ Special fried rice etc.

✖ Crispy duck with pancakes

✖ Fried spring rolls, won-ton, king prawns etc.

✖ Sweet and sour dishes in which the pork, prawns or chicken have been fried in batter

✖ Sweet desserts

✔ CHOOSE:

✔ Steamed dim sum

✔ Boiled or steamed rice

✔ Glutinous rice

✔ Stir-fried vegetables, prawns, chicken etc.

✔ Spicy hot Szechuan dishes

Travel tips; Surviving your holiday

We all look forward to our holidays and, for many of us, they are the incentive to slim down so that we can don a bikini on the beach. However, the sad truth is that most of us return home heavier than when we set out, and have to go on another diet to shed the pounds we put on during a fortnight in the sun. Here are some tips to help you avoid putting on weight and return even fitter and slimmer than you were before your departure.

If you are self-catering
■ Pack your scales and measuring spoons, sweeteners and skimmed powdered milk. Don't guesstimate food weights and volumes.
■ Discover the local markets and experiment with fresh fruit and vegetables.
■ Look forward to just one main meal a day. At other times, eat light meals or snacks, e.g. fresh fruit and vegetables.

If you stay in a hotel
■ In buffet meals limit yourself to one plate (not piled high) and one trip. Don't go up for second helpings.
■ Make sure at least half of the food on your plate is fruit or vegetables.

General tips
■ Limit ice creams to one a day.
■ Avoid the local freshly baked crusty bread unless you can stop at one piece.
■ Drink sugar-free drinks or sparkling water
■ Only drink alcohol if you can stop at two drinks.
■ Exercise every day: swim in the pool, go for a walk or a cycle, try watersports, tennis or golf.

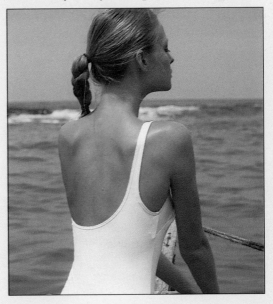

FAST FOODS

It is very convenient to grab a 'fast food' when you're feeling hungry, but unfortunately many of them are fried or high in fat, and loaded with unwanted calories. The healthiest fast food that you can eat is probably a sandwich; for low-calorie ideas, turn to pages 54-55.

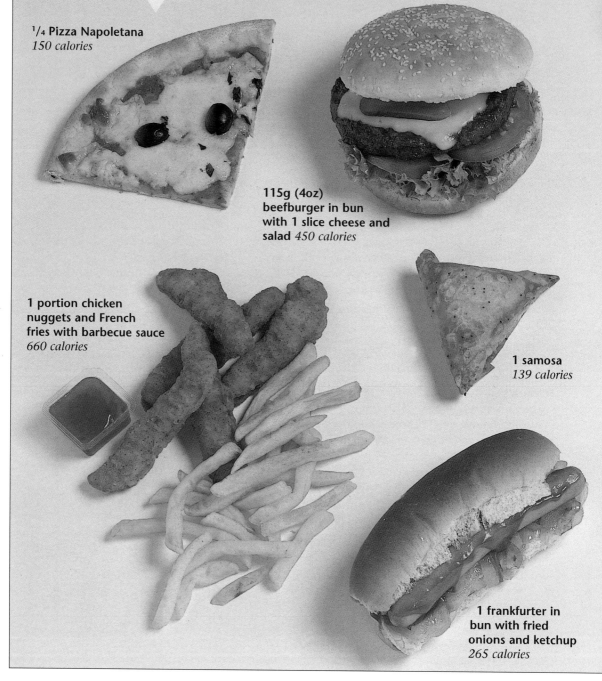

¹/₄ Pizza Napoletana
150 calories

115g (4oz) beefburger in bun with 1 slice cheese and salad *450 calories*

1 portion chicken nuggets and French fries with barbecue sauce
660 calories

1 samosa
139 calories

1 frankfurter in bun with fried onions and ketchup
265 calories

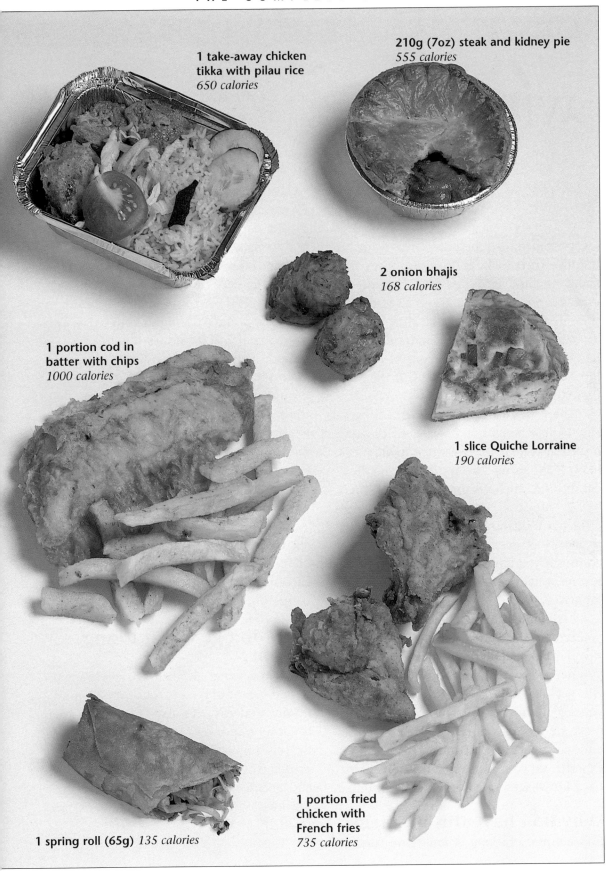

**1 take-away chicken
tikka with pilau rice**
650 calories

210g (7oz) steak and kidney pie
555 calories

2 onion bhajis
168 calories

**1 portion cod in
batter with chips**
1000 calories

1 slice Quiche Lorraine
190 calories

1 spring roll (65g) *135 calories*

**1 portion fried
chicken with
French fries**
735 calories

WHY DIET?

Most women diet because they want to improve their looks and the way they feel about themselves. This isn't because of pressure from the media; this is a self-driven pressure to be the person that they want to be. When you lose weight, you immediately feel that at last you are in control of your life – and that control begins with the food that you eat every day.

There are many good reasons why you should lose weight, not least of all your health. If you are overweight, you are more likely to suffer from many medical conditions, such as heart disease, high blood pressure, diabetes, strokes and arthritis. And treatment of these conditions is more complex and more difficult to control if you are overweight. However, by losing weight, these conditions can be improved.

At Slimmer Clubs UK, our aim is to help you achieve the weight that is right for you. If you decide to join one of our local classes you needn't worry about the reception you will get – nobody is going to make fun of you or humiliate you. Instead, you will make new friends and discover reassuring and supportive people who have experienced your problems themselves and have lost weight successfully with our diet.

Why do I have this problem?

It is tempting to look at your slim friends and ask the million-dollar question: "Why can't I look like them?" The simple answer is, of course, that you can. It is true that some lucky people seem to be able to eat anything and everything and still lose weight or stay slim, but this is not the norm for the average dieter. It is a simple fact that if you consume more calories than your body needs, those extra calories are stored in your body as fat. Eat less calories than your body needs and you will lose weight.

You need to consume 3,500 calories to gain one pound of weight; conversely, you need to eat 3,500 calories less to lose one pound. This is why sensible dieting can seem such a slow process. Seasoned dieters have all sorts of excuses to explain why they cannot lose weight, but glandular problems are rare, heavier people have a higher metabolic rate than their slim friends, and fatness is not hereditary although bad eating habits may be handed down from one generation to the next.

Now is the time to throw all these excuses out of the window. If you follow the diet in this book, you will lose weight. How successful you will be is entirely in your hands, and only you can do it.

How do I go about losing weight?

Once you have decided to lose weight, impatience often sets in. We all want instant and easy results – to be slim and beautiful tomorrow. Although we may look for that non-existent miracle cure, there is no diet where you can eat whatever you like and still lose weight fast. It is from this irrational thinking that fad diets are created.

The only sensible way to lose weight is

QUIZ: WHAT SORT OF DIETER ARE YOU?

Answer the questions honestly to find out what sort of dieter you are, and then turn to page 109.

1 Which breakfast would you most like to eat on a diet?
(a) By and large, I have the same breakfast every day. ☑
(b) Bread or toast with jam. ☐
(c) I eat breakfast when the family has left in the morning. ☐
(d) A cooked breakfast if possible. ☐
(e) No, I wouldn't eat breakfast. ☐

2 You're hungry and it's 11 o'clock. What do you reach for?
(a) A piece of fruit. ☐
(b) A low-calorie chocolate bar. ☐
(c) That cream cake at the back of the fridge left over from last night. ☐
(d) You plan to have only one biscuit but this may lead to more. ☐
(e) Nothing. ☑

3 You go into the supermarket to grab something for lunch. Which do you choose?
(a) The lowest low-calorie sandwiches? ☑
(b) Cottage cheese and salad plus a wicked low-calorie chocolate dessert. ☐
(c) A low-calorie sandwich plus a family bag of crisps for later. ☐
(d) Anything you fancy because you've had a stressful morning. ☐
(e) A piece of fruit or a diet yogurt. ☐

4 It's 4 o'clock and you're feeling a bit peckish. What do you have?
(a) Vegetable crudités and a low-calorie dip you prepared earlier. ☐
(b) A cup of tea and a kit-kat. ☐
(c) Something out of the fridge while there's no-one around. ☐
(d) One of the chocolate mini-rolls in the packet you bought earlier. ☐
(e) Nothing. ☐

5 You're eating your evening meal with the rest of the family. Which would you choose?
(a) A healthy, low-fat meal for all of you? ☐
(b) Do you make sure you leave plenty of room for your pudding? ☐
(c) Do you resist the potatoes and bread but perhaps eat them later? ☐
(d) Are you careful with the main course but demolish the dessert? ☐
(e) Do you eat a different low-calorie meal to the rest of the family? ☑

6 Bedtime approaches and hunger pangs reappear. What do you do?
(a) You say to yourself: "Do I really want something? I'm not really hungry so I'll have a bath instead." ☑
(b) Look for that elusive mini-chocolate treat left over from the children's lunch box. ☐
(c) Make an excuse to get a cup of tea – and raid the biscuit tin. ☐
(d) You eat the family packet of crisps you bought at lunchtime. ☐
(e) Have nothing. ☐

7 You're eating out in your favourite restaurant. What do you choose?
(a) Enjoy all three courses, choosing low-calorie dishes. ☐
(b) Choose a low-calorie starter and main course and reward yourself for being good with a creamy pudding. ☑
(c) Choose three low-calorie courses and then eat the Mars Bar in the fridge at home before going to bed. ☐
(d) Anything and everything. You'll restart the diet on Monday. ☐
(e) Skip the starter and dessert – just have a main course and salad. ☐

8 You're doing your weekly shop. What do you put in your trolley? ☑
(a) Lots of fruit and vegetables, and healthy low-calorie foods. ☑
(b) You're careful all the way round until you succumb to the aromas of the fresh bakery counter. ☐
(c) A pick n' mix bag of sweets 'for the children' which is put in the glove compartment of the car. ☐
(d) You hide the six-pack of chocolate bars underneath the vegetables. ☐
(e) As little as possible. ☐

9 You've started a diet and an exercise programme. Which of the following most resembles you?
(a) You build up gradually to three 20-minute sessions per week and eat sensibly. ☑
(b) You enrol at your local sports centre but notice there is a poolside café with a selection of sweet treats with which to reward yourself. ☐
(c) You attend your local aerobics class with a chocolate bar hidden in your bag to restore your energy level. ☐
(d) Life is too busy and stressful to exercise regularly, but guilt drives you to the biscuit tin. ☐
(e) You work out for 30 minutes five times a week with just a bottle of mineral water to sustain you. ☐

10 You've been dieting for three weeks and your weight loss has ground to a halt. What do you do?
(a) Accept that this is perfectly normal and stick with it. ☑
(b) Console yourself with a cream cake. ☐
(c) Tell your partner you've lost weight anyway. ☐
(d) Your frustration grows: it's time to devour the contents of the fridge. ☐
(e) Starve those extra pounds off. ☐

(A) 6
(B) 1
(C) 0
(D) 0
(E) 3

to change your eating habits in a way that will not make you feel deprived, and will allow you to lose a steady one-and-a-half to two pounds a week. The diets in this book are approved by doctors, and will ensure that you lose weight slowly and safely without damaging your health. By adopting healthier eating habits, you will establish a new diet for life which will help you to maintain your new weight in the future. Set yourself some realistic targets to encourage you to stick to your diet.

■ **Target One:** Take one day at a time – just plan to follow your diet today and tomorrow will take care of itself.

■ **Target Two:** Start exercising and build up gradually so that you exercise for a minimum of three 20-minute sessions per week. Weight loss is about burning up calories as well as dieting.

■ **Target Three:** Set yourself a realistic weight loss goal – successful results are measured both in will power and sheer determination, not time. If your weight built up slowly over many months or even years, it will not disappear overnight.

How can I stick to my diet longer than a day?

Starting a diet is easy, but it's a well-known fact that most diets start on Monday, only to fail at best by Friday, and at worst by Monday afternoon! This is because we see weekends as a time for relaxation and as well as forgetting about work and the daily routine, we often relax our eating habits and indulge, usually excessively, in the foods that give us pleasure. Unfortunately, these are often the most calorie-laden ones. However, you can still enjoy weekends when you are losing weight on our diet, and

even eat out in your favourite restaurant.

If dieting during the week is a problem, you need to look at the dieting challenges you face every day. You will probably find that the foods you eat are determined by your timetable at work or at home. For example, perhaps you are used to having a biscuit with your morning coffee; if so, substitute a lower-calorie piece of fruit, or avoid the kitchen or works canteen around 11 o'clock. If you have small children, then 4.00pm may be a difficult time when you are preparing the children's tea. You need to plan your tactics for these times – keep a diet yogurt handy in the fridge or a fresh fruit salad or some raw vegetables with a low-calorie dip.

Whatever your difficult time you can and will overcome it. It will take time to adapt your eating habits but once you have learnt the skills of sensible eating, long-term weight loss and maintenance will be easy.

I've lost and put weight back on before – how will it be different this time?

Long-term weight maintenance is a skill that you can learn. Most dieters know only too well how to lose weight but maintaining the weight loss is more of a challenge. When you start your diet, it will help if you tell yourself this really is the last time ever.

Wouldn't it be wonderful to know that you will never again have to motivate yourself to start another diet? The way to achieving this success is to change the way you think and feel about food. If we only ate when we were hungry, none of us would

Continued on page 108

SUCCESS STORY ✓

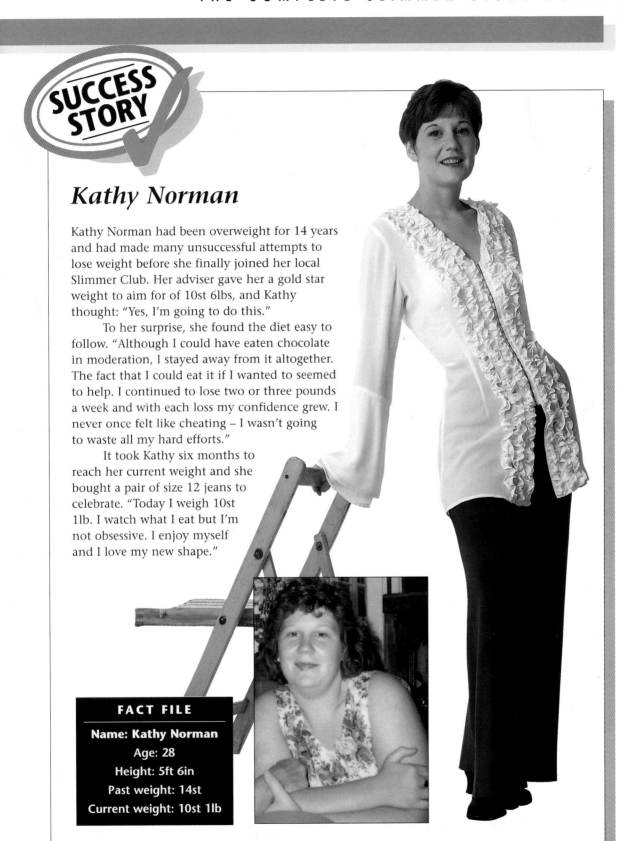

Kathy Norman

Kathy Norman had been overweight for 14 years and had made many unsuccessful attempts to lose weight before she finally joined her local Slimmer Club. Her adviser gave her a gold star weight to aim for of 10st 6lbs, and Kathy thought: "Yes, I'm going to do this."

To her surprise, she found the diet easy to follow. "Although I could have eaten chocolate in moderation, I stayed away from it altogether. The fact that I could eat it if I wanted to seemed to help. I continued to lose two or three pounds a week and with each loss my confidence grew. I never once felt like cheating – I wasn't going to waste all my hard efforts."

It took Kathy six months to reach her current weight and she bought a pair of size 12 jeans to celebrate. "Today I weigh 10st 1lb. I watch what I eat but I'm not obsessive. I enjoy myself and I love my new shape."

FACT FILE
Name: Kathy Norman
Age: 28
Height: 5ft 6in
Past weight: 14st
Current weight: 10st 1lb

DRINKS AND NIBBLES

Beware of party drinks and nibbles, as this photoguide shows. You are safest sticking to low-calorie diet drinks and mixers or unsweetened fruit juice. To make wine go further and reduce calories, you can top it up with sparkling mineral water for a delicious spritzer.

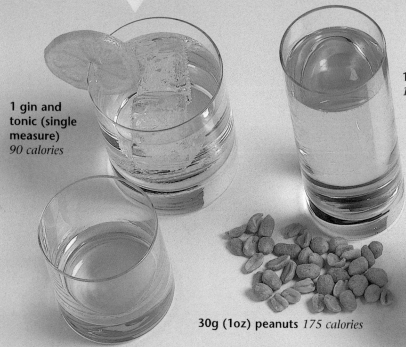

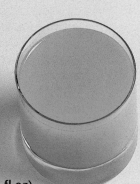

1 spritzer
115 calories

2 mini quiches (30g each)
170 calories

1 gin and tonic (single measure)
90 calories

30g (1oz) peanuts *175 calories*

1 whisky (single measure)
50 calories

115ml (4 fl oz) unsweetened orange juice
49 calories

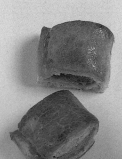

2 mini sausage rolls
90 calories

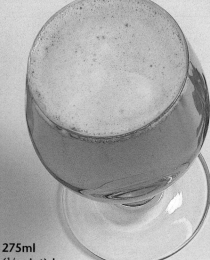

275ml (¹/₂ pint) lager
90 calories

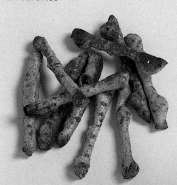

15g (¹/₂ oz) twiglets
60 calories

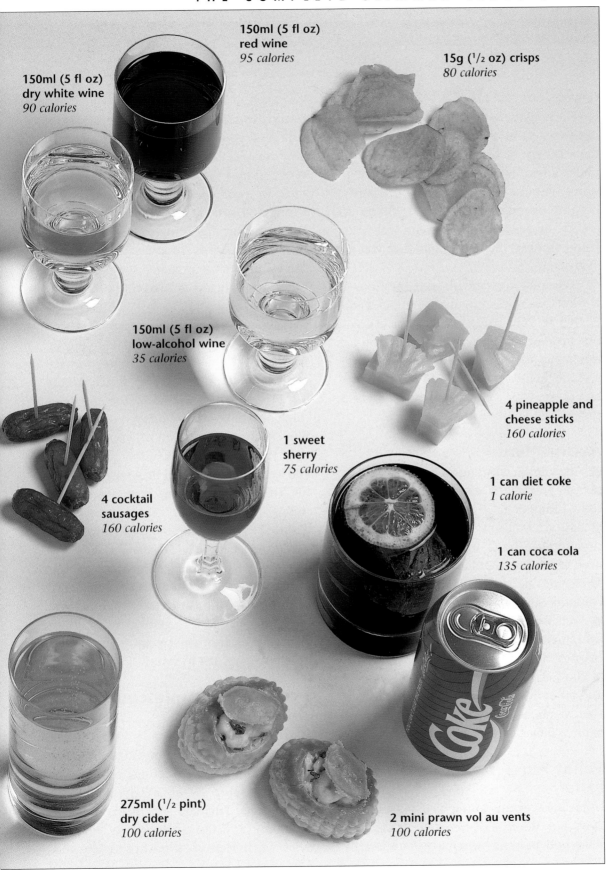

**150ml (5 fl oz)
red wine**
95 calories

15g (¹/₂ oz) crisps
80 calories

**150ml (5 fl oz)
dry white wine**
90 calories

**150ml (5 fl oz)
low-alcohol wine**
35 calories

**4 pineapple and
cheese sticks**
160 calories

**1 sweet
sherry**
75 calories

**4 cocktail
sausages**
160 calories

1 can diet coke
1 calorie

1 can coca cola
135 calories

**275ml (¹/₂ pint)
dry cider**
100 calories

2 mini prawn vol au vents
100 calories

Continued from page 104
have a weight problem. However, eating is not just a solution for hunger, and we eat for a variety of reasons: when we are sad, under stress, upset, celebrating, bored, or simply because we just enjoy food. There is nothing wrong with this, but if you do eat for any of these reasons and not just when you're hungry, then it is likely that you are overweight.

Learning to cope with your emotions in a way that does not involve food is the answer to your success. Eating a cake will not make your anger disappear; if you are miserable, it will just add to your misery and the inches on your hips! You must have tactics up your sleeve to cope with these times. Try the following:

Action plan

■ Ask yourself why you are feeling this way.
■ Ask yourself if eating will make this feeling diminish.
■ Distract yourself from the threatening situation: go for a walk, take a hot bath even if it's the afternoon, phone a friend. These are all preferable to admiring the contents of the biscuit tin.
■ Wait for 10 minutes, and if the desire to eat remains, have something that is low in calories.
■ If all else fails, eat what you are craving and enjoy it! Maybe next time you will be able to rescue yourself from the situation before you get this far down in the plan.

What happens if I go off the rails?

In an ideal world, losing weight would be easy, but don't fool yourself. Inevitably, there will be times when you temporarily lose control of the foods you eat. Don't worry – this is quite normal. The success or failure of your diet will be determined by how you feel mentally about losing weight. When things are going well, it is easy to stick to your diet, but when things go wrong and you are busy or under pressure, you are most likely to stray. Recognising this in advance is your first step towards success; if you are prepared for the difficult times, you can rest assured that you will be able to cope.

Step two is to use any set-back as a lesson learned. If you have temporarily 'blown' your diet, ask yourself why. What was the trigger that sent you off in search of the biscuit tin? When you know the answer to this, you will be better equipped to cope next time. A common reaction when people blow their diets is to throw caution to the wind and carry on eating until they have had their fill. This is bingeing, and it always leads to feelings of guilt, which are then followed by the need to cheer yourself up with more food – thus the vicious circle begins.

If you go off the rails, stop yourself before you go too far and put the experience behind you. You can't correct the damage but you can stop it getting worse. Take tomorrow as another day and plan to stick rigidly to your diet in future.

I've reached a plateau – what can I do?

Many dieters experience a rapid initial weight loss in the first week or two, but then it slows down, sometimes to the point when they stop losing weight despite all their efforts. This is a weight loss plateau, but with a little perseverance you can overcome it. Here are some tips to help you:

- Stick to the exact quantities stated in your diet. Measure food accurately and don't guesstimate.
- You must eat all your allowances every day. Do not drink or eat anything that is not included in the diet.
- Drink plenty of water.
- If you are hungry between meals nibble low-calorie vegetables.
- Don't give up and start bingeing or comfort eating. Stick with it and you *will* lose weight.
- Eat less fat calories – it is easier to burn carbohydrate ones.
- Step up your level of exercise.

Finally, be kind to yourself

Dieting is a challenge, and there will be difficult times but remember that you really can be successful and lose weight. No-one expects you to stick to the diet 100 per cent all the time – human nature prevents us being perfect. However, being hard on yourself may actually stop you being successful. Learn to like yourself for what you are, set-backs included, and this extra self-esteem will give you the confidence you need to see you through the good times and the bad.

HOW DID YOU SCORE?

A Mostly 'a' answers: The sensible dieter
Well done. You're dieting sensibly and you will achieve long-term slow, sensible weight loss, and will find it easy to maintain your target weight.

B Mostly 'b' answers: The sweet tooth dieter
Your sweet tooth makes dieting difficult at times. Don't worry; you can still be successful if you keep it under control and enjoy sweets in moderation.

C Mostly 'c' answers: The secret eater
The chances are that you are a secret eater. You're an angel when surrounded by family and friends but blow your diet when you're alone. It will help if you share this secret with someone

close so that they can be supportive and help you change your habits.

D Mostly 'd' answers: The binger
You may sometimes find that in moments of weakness you turn to food in a big way. Bingeing means different things to different people, but it's never going to help you lose weight successfully. It's now time to look at the situations that make you binge, and set about changing your habits for ever.

E Mostly 'e' answers: The crash dieter
You're definitely an 'all or nothing' person. In your eyes, dieting has to be painful to work. But stop and think! How many times have you been down this road before? Long-term success will only be yours if you eat and diet sensibly.

BREADS AND PASTRIES

These are many a dieter's downfall and need to be controlled carefully, especially cakes and pastries. Crispbreads and mini pittas make a low-calorie light lunch when eaten with salad and some lean meat, chicken, fish or cottage cheese.

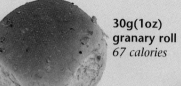

30g(1oz) granary roll
67 calories

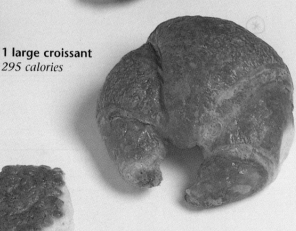

1 dairy cream chocolate éclair
175 calories

1 medium-cut slice white bread
80 calories

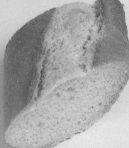

1 large croissant
295 calories

30g (1oz) slice French bread
80 calories

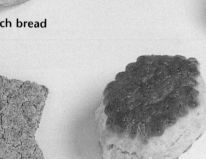

60g (2oz) jam doughnut
250 calories

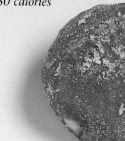

45g (1¹/₂oz) Devon scone
183 calories

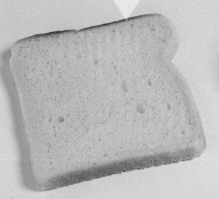

2 crispbreads
50 calories

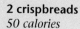

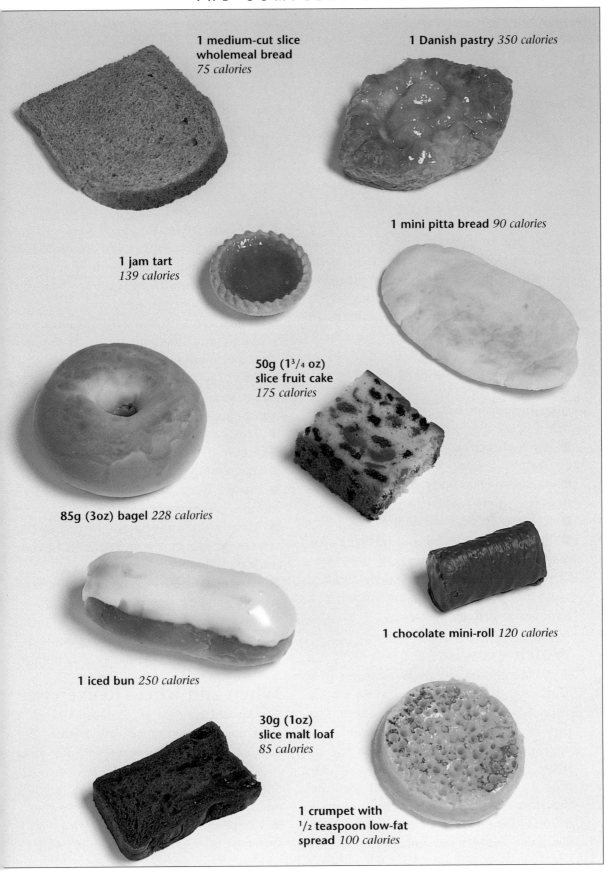

1 medium-cut slice wholemeal bread *75 calories*

1 Danish pastry *350 calories*

1 mini pitta bread *90 calories*

1 jam tart *139 calories*

50g (1³/₄ oz) slice fruit cake *175 calories*

85g (3oz) bagel *228 calories*

1 chocolate mini-roll *120 calories*

1 iced bun *250 calories*

30g (1oz) slice malt loaf *85 calories*

1 crumpet with ¹/₂ teaspoon low-fat spread *100 calories*

Exercise

Regular exercise will help to speed up your weight loss by burning up excess calories which are stored in your body as fat. It will tone up and firm those problem areas like hips and thighs, help you lose inches off your waist and flatten your stomach. In fact, the benefits of exercise are seemingly endless.

■ It makes you fitter and healthier.

■ It improves your circulation and strengthens your heart and lungs, thereby reducing the risk of heart disease.

■ It refreshes your mind, relieves tension and helps you relax.

■ It makes your body more supple and flexible.

■ It speeds up your metabolism.

■ It gives you a sense of well-being and makes you feel younger.

What's more, exercise is enjoyable and fun – and it's never too late to start, even if you have never exercised before.

Which exercise?

If you are unused to exercise, start off in a gentle way. You might like to go for a brisk walk each day – perhaps to the shops, the park or round the block. You could join your local gym or exercise class, cycle or swim, or try out our home work-out (see page 114) which has been designed by fitness expert Diana Moran. The important thing is to enjoy the exercise you choose; if you don't, then try something else.

Exercise safely

It is very important that you always follow our basic safety guidelines if you are to enjoy the benefits of exercise without getting stiff, sore or injured.

■ Train, don't strain. Ease into exercise gradually and build up slowly as you get fitter and more supple.

■ Don't 'go for the burn'. Stretch only as far as feels comfortable. If it hurts, stop immediately.

■ Check with your doctor before you start, especially if you have a medical condition or are carrying a lot of excess weight.

■ Always warm-up thoroughly for 10-15 minutes before you exercise.

■ Always do some cool-down stretches after exercising to ease and stretch out your muscles and prevent stiffness.

■ Wear some loose comfortable clothing or a leotard and proper training shoes.

■ Always move carefully and rhythmically – don't make sudden, jerky movements.

■ Never exercise immediately after a meal.

When and where to exercise

You should exercise at least three times a week for a minimum of 20 minutes per session. Try to build exercise into your regular routine so that it becomes an enjoyable habit that you wouldn't miss for anything. Here are some tips to help you:

■ Exercise at every opportunity, e.g. climb the stairs instead of taking the lift; walk to

the shops or to school instead of driving.
■ Never drive if you can walk or cycle instead.
■ Make exercise a family activity at weekends, e.g. walking, cycling, swimming.

Our home work-out

The work-out on the following pages has been created by Diana Moran and she is featured within it with two successful slimmers who have both lost weight with Slimmer Clubs UK – Sarah Bingham and Jill Lawrence (see pages 44-45).

The work-out has three parts: the warm-up exercises; stretching and toning exercises; and cool-down stretches. We have not included any aerobic exercises as we feel that it is a good idea if you attain a basic level of fitness before you embark on these.

Diana recommends that you start by doing eight repetitions of each exercise. However, if you find a particular exercise very difficult, then you can decrease the repetitions from eight to four, and then increase them gradually as you get fitter.

If you want to work on a specific problem area, such as your stomach or your thighs, increase the repetitions from eight to sixteen. As your fitness improves, increase the repetitions. However, do not over-do it; it is better to come back to that area later on in your work-out and then do another eight repetitions.

Aerobic exercise

This helps improve your heart and lung efficiency and builds up stamina. If you want to introduce an aerobic element into your personal exercise programme, you could try one of the following:
■ Jogging on the spot.

■ Cycling on the road or an exercise bike.
■ Swimming.
■ Brisk walking.
■ Skipping.
■ Stepping up and down off a stair or low stool.
■ Dancing to your favourite music.
■ Exercising on a rowing machine.
■ Jogging outside, preferably on grass – not on the road or hard pavements.

These are all excellent forms of aerobic exercise and should be performed for 10-20 minutes three times a week.

Fitness expert Diana Moran

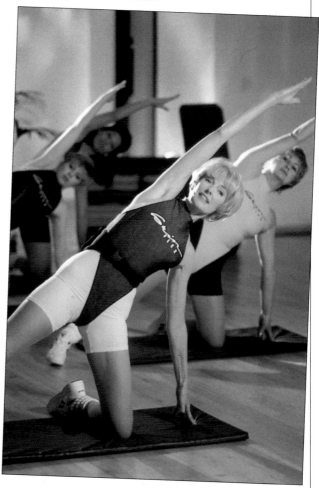

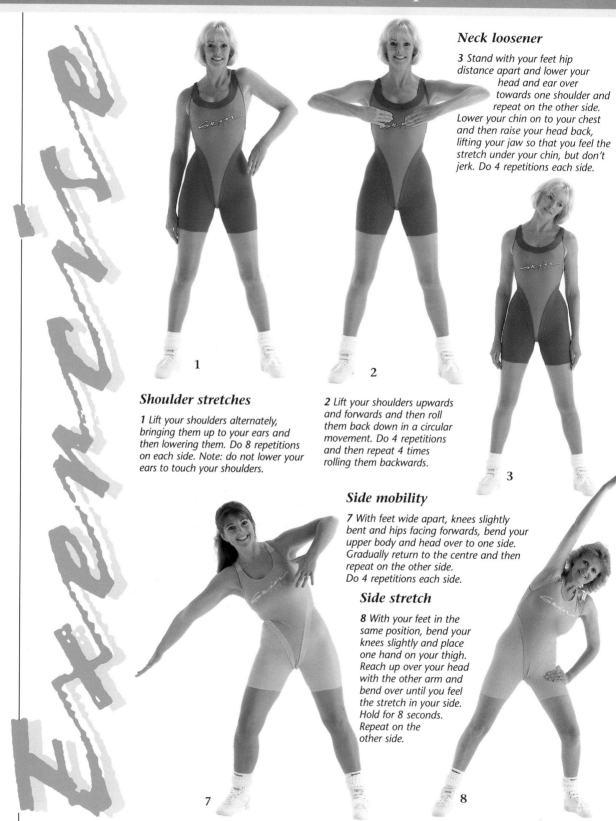

Neck loosener

3 Stand with your feet hip distance apart and lower your head and ear over towards one shoulder and repeat on the other side. Lower your chin on to your chest and then raise your head back, lifting your jaw so that you feel the stretch under your chin, but don't jerk. Do 4 repetitions each side.

Shoulder stretches

1 Lift your shoulders alternately, bringing them up to your ears and then lowering them. Do 8 repetitions on each side. Note: do not lower your ears to touch your shoulders.

2 Lift your shoulders upwards and forwards and then roll them back down in a circular movement. Do 4 repetitions and then repeat 4 times rolling them backwards.

Side mobility

7 With feet wide apart, knees slightly bent and hips facing forwards, bend your upper body and head over to one side. Gradually return to the centre and then repeat on the other side. Do 4 repetitions each side.

Side stretch

8 With your feet in the same position, bend your knees slightly and place one hand on your thigh. Reach up over your head with the other arm and bend over until you feel the stretch in your side. Hold for 8 seconds. Repeat on the other side.

Upper body mobility

4 Stand with feet shoulder width apart and knees slightly bent, hips facing forwards and stomach pulled in. With your arms held in front of you at shoulder height, twist the upper body to the left, then to the centre, and then to the right. Repeat 4 times. Be sure to move only the upper body from the waist up; keep the hips facing forwards.

5 With your feet slightly wider apart and knees bent, swing your arms rhythmically from side to side, lowering them as they cross your body. Transfer your weight from foot to foot as you do so and don't bend forwards or backwards. Repeat 8 times.

6 With feet shoulder width apart, reach up with one arm over your head as high as possible. Repeat with the other arm. Do 8 repetitions each side.

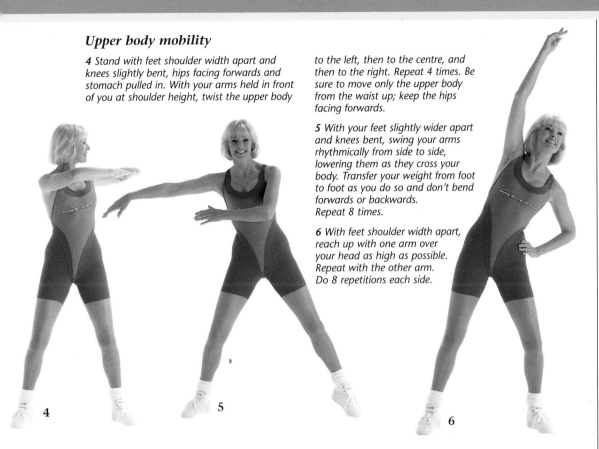

4

5

6

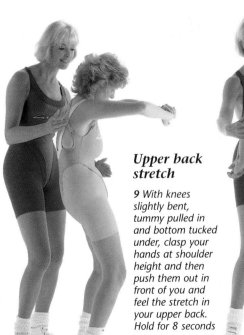

Upper back stretch

9 With knees slightly bent, tummy pulled in and bottom tucked under, clasp your hands at shoulder height and then push them out in front of you and feel the stretch in your upper back. Hold for 8 seconds

10

Chest stretch

10 From the same position, clasp your hands behind you and then pull your shoulders back without arching your back. Hold for 8 seconds.

Upper arm stretch

11 Put one hand behind your neck with the fingers pointing downwards into the small of your back. Take your other arm over your head and rest the fingers on your elbow, easing it back and down until you feel the stretch in your upper arm. Repeat on the other side. Hold for 8 seconds.

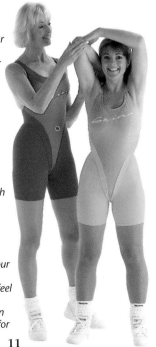

11

Foot and ankle mobilizers

1 Stretch one leg out in front of you with your heel on the floor. The knee of your supporting leg should be slightly bent. Now bring your foot back as close to your supporting leg as possible and point your toes. Repeat 8 times and then do 8 repetitions on the other side.

2 With your toes facing forwards, slowly raise and lower yourself on your toes 8 times. Do not roll forwards or backwards.

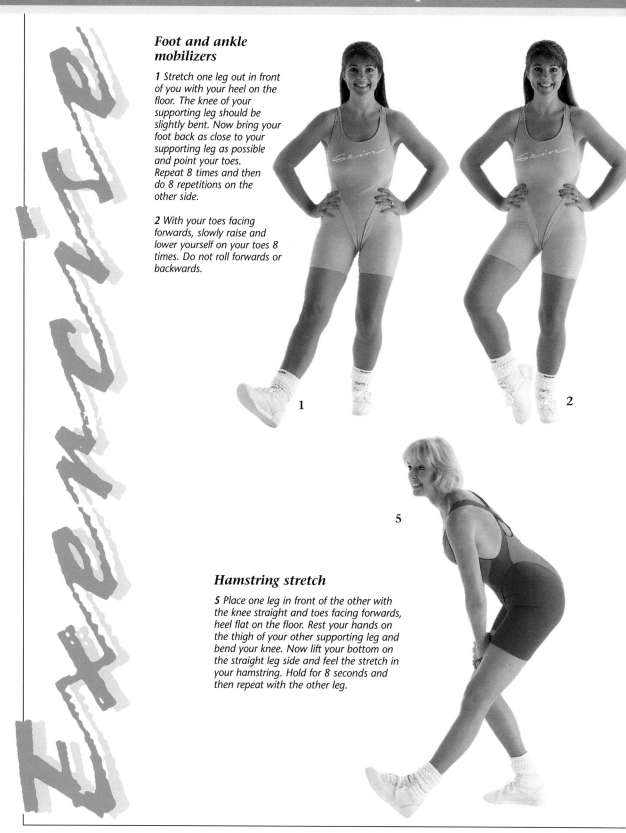

1

2

5

Hamstring stretch

5 Place one leg in front of the other with the knee straight and toes facing forwards, heel flat on the floor. Rest your hands on the thigh of your other supporting leg and bend your knee. Now lift your bottom on the straight leg side and feel the stretch in your hamstring. Hold for 8 seconds and then repeat with the other leg.

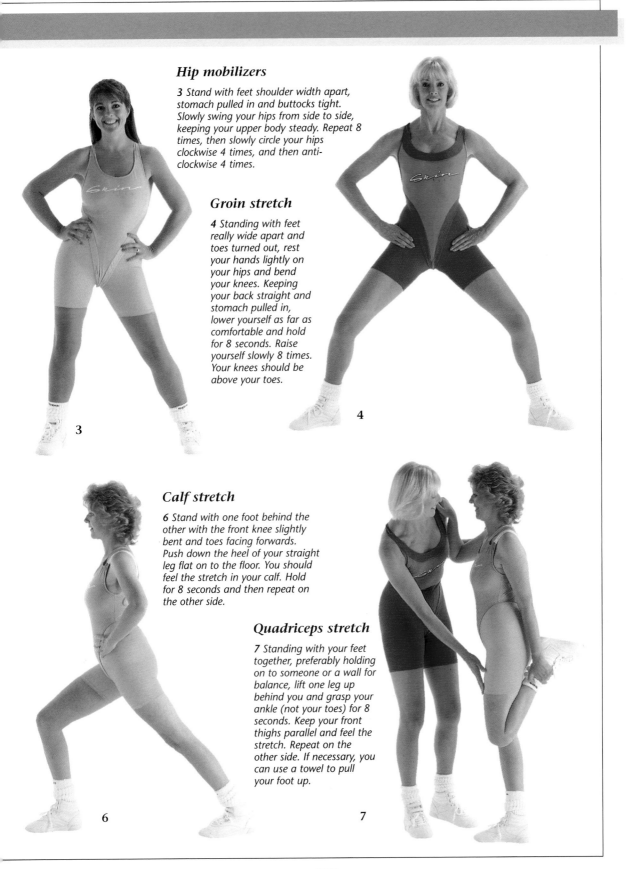

Hip mobilizers

3 Stand with feet shoulder width apart, stomach pulled in and buttocks tight. Slowly swing your hips from side to side, keeping your upper body steady. Repeat 8 times, then slowly circle your hips clockwise 4 times, and then anti-clockwise 4 times.

Groin stretch

4 Standing with feet really wide apart and toes turned out, rest your hands lightly on your hips and bend your knees. Keeping your back straight and stomach pulled in, lower yourself as far as comfortable and hold for 8 seconds. Raise yourself slowly 8 times. Your knees should be above your toes.

Calf stretch

6 Stand with one foot behind the other with the front knee slightly bent and toes facing forwards. Push down the heel of your straight leg flat on to the floor. You should feel the stretch in your calf. Hold for 8 seconds and then repeat on the other side.

Quadriceps stretch

7 Standing with your feet together, preferably holding on to someone or a wall for balance, lift one leg up behind you and grasp your ankle (not your toes) for 8 seconds. Keep your front thighs parallel and feel the stretch. Repeat on the other side. If necessary, you can use a towel to pull your foot up.

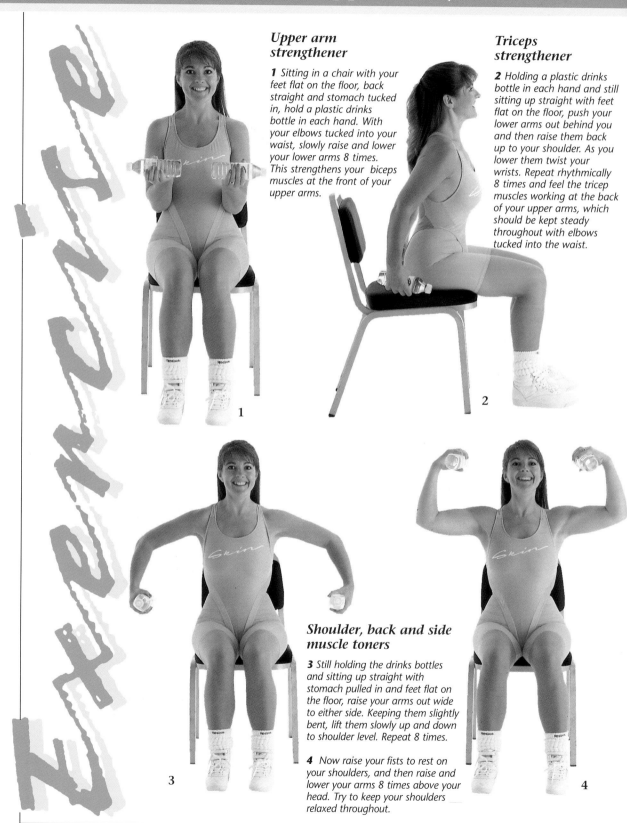

Upper arm strengthener

1 Sitting in a chair with your feet flat on the floor, back straight and stomach tucked in, hold a plastic drinks bottle in each hand. With your elbows tucked into your waist, slowly raise and lower your lower arms 8 times. This strengthens your biceps muscles at the front of your upper arms.

Triceps strengthener

2 Holding a plastic drinks bottle in each hand and still sitting up straight with feet flat on the floor, push your lower arms out behind you and then raise them back up to your shoulder. As you lower them twist your wrists. Repeat rhythmically 8 times and feel the tricep muscles working at the back of your upper arms, which should be kept steady throughout with elbows tucked into the waist.

Shoulder, back and side muscle toners

3 Still holding the drinks bottles and sitting up straight with stomach pulled in and feet flat on the floor, raise your arms out wide to either side. Keeping them slightly bent, lift them slowly up and down to shoulder level. Repeat 8 times.

4 Now raise your fists to rest on your shoulders, and then raise and lower your arms 8 times above your head. Try to keep your shoulders relaxed throughout.

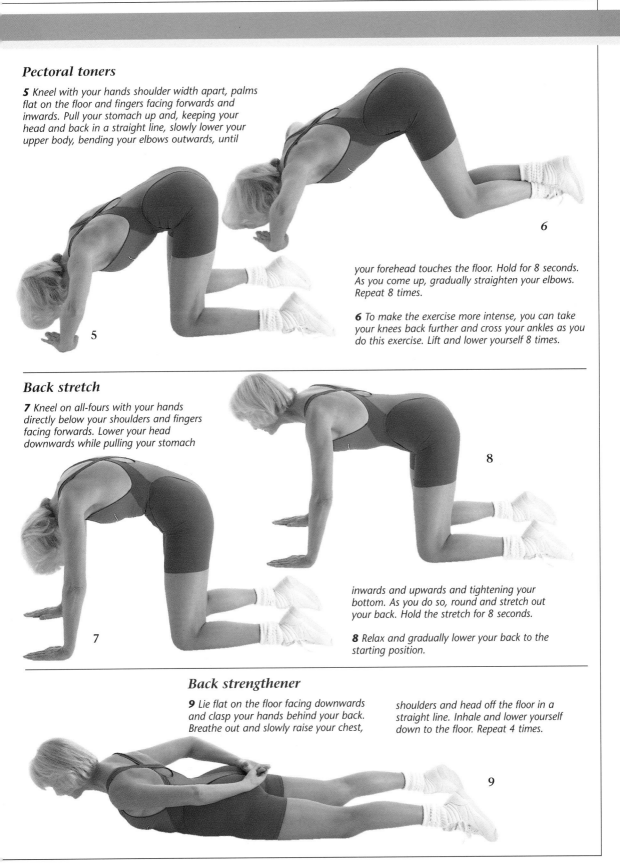

Pectoral toners

5 Kneel with your hands shoulder width apart, palms flat on the floor and fingers facing forwards and inwards. Pull your stomach up and, keeping your head and back in a straight line, slowly lower your upper body, bending your elbows outwards, until

your forehead touches the floor. Hold for 8 seconds. As you come up, gradually straighten your elbows. Repeat 8 times.

6 To make the exercise more intense, you can take your knees back further and cross your ankles as you do this exercise. Lift and lower yourself 8 times.

Back stretch

7 Kneel on all-fours with your hands directly below your shoulders and fingers facing forwards. Lower your head downwards while pulling your stomach

inwards and upwards and tightening your bottom. As you do so, round and stretch out your back. Hold the stretch for 8 seconds.

8 Relax and gradually lower your back to the starting position.

Back strengthener

9 Lie flat on the floor facing downwards and clasp your hands behind your back. Breathe out and slowly raise your chest, shoulders and head off the floor in a straight line. Inhale and lower yourself down to the floor. Repeat 4 times.

Pelvic tilt

1 Lie flat on the floor with knees and feet shoulder width apart and hands resting lightly on your stomach. As you breathe in, press your lower back and waist down on to the floor. This tips your pelvis upwards and forwards. Repeat 8 times. This gives you central control and is the basis of all the abdominal exercises.

Sit-ups

2 Lie down with knees bent and feet flat on the floor, resting your hands on your thighs. Keeping your stomach pulled in, exhale and slide your hands up your thighs towards your knees, raising your head and shoulders off the ground. Inhale and slowly slide your hands back and lower yourself. Repeat 8 times.

3 Still in the same position, place your fingertips lightly on either side of your head with elbows out to the sides as far back as possible. Exhale and lift your head and shoulders off the ground slowly and rhythmically. Lower them and repeat 8 times.

4 With one elbow on the floor, your fingertips resting on your head, lift your head and shoulders off the floor and stretch out your hand to touch the opposite knee. As you do so, twist your shoulder over. Inhale and relax. Repeat 8 times.

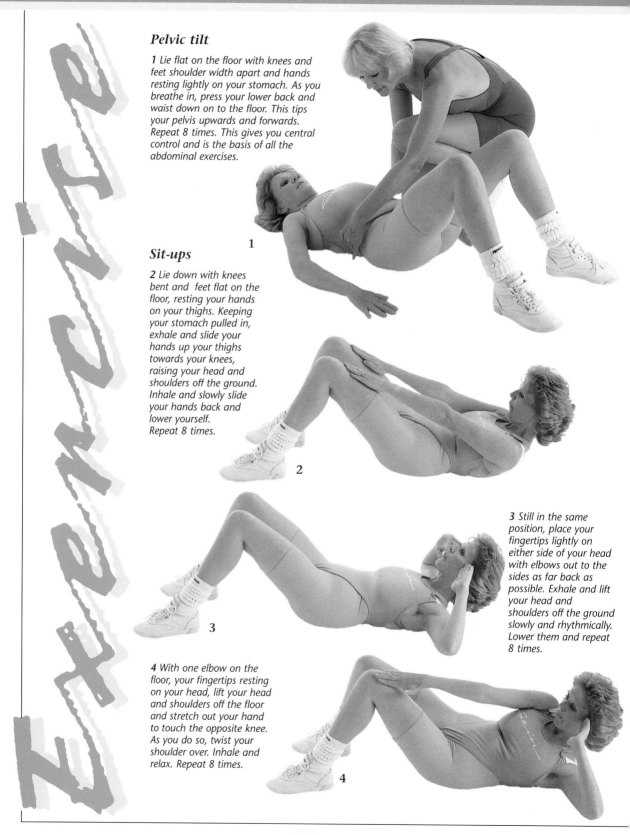

Criss-cross abdominal strengthener

5 Lie on the floor with knees bent and bend one elbow and rest your fingers on the sides of your head. Cross your knee on the same side over the other one. Exhale and lift your other arm, raising your head and shoulders off the floor, reaching across with your elbow to touch the outside of your bent knee. Inhale and relax. Repeat 8 times on each side.

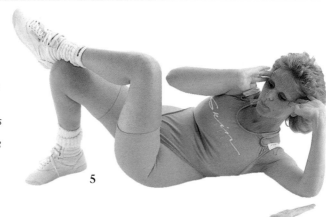

5

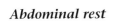

6

Abdominal rest

6 To rest your abdominal muscles in between exercises, lie on your back with your knees bent and your lower back pressed into the floor. Slowly sweep each arm alternately up off the floor and over your head, just touching your ears. Repeat 4 times.

Bottom tightener

7 Stand holding on to the back of a chair for support. With stomach and bottom pulled in, stretch one leg back behind you with the toes resting on the floor. Slowly lift and lower this leg, keeping it straight, for 8 repetitions. Bend the support leg slightly Repeat with the other leg. You should feel the muscles in your bottom working.

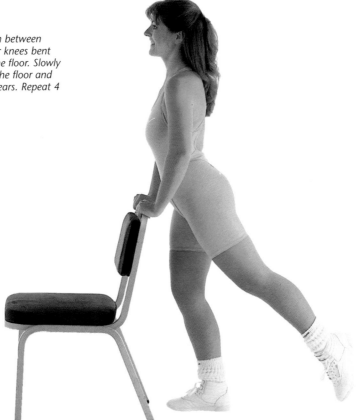

7

Outer thigh toners

1 Lie on your side with bent elbow and resting your head on one hand. Use your other hand to support your body. Bend your knees back, keeping thighs and upper body in a straight line. With stomach pulled in and buttocks tight, raise your bent upper leg slowly and then lower it to the floor 8 times. Keep your knees parallel,

feet flexed and don't roll forward or back. Repeat 8 times on the other side.

2 To make the exercise harder, you can lie as before with your lower leg bent back and raise your upper leg straight out with foot flexed. Repeat 8 times on each side.

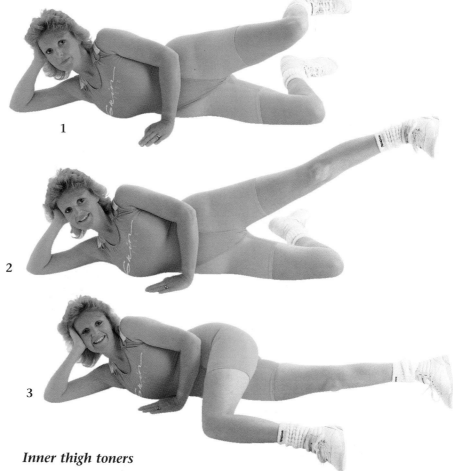

Inner thigh toners

3 Lie as before but place your top leg over your lower leg with your knee on the floor for support. With foot flexed, as before, raise your lower leg slowly up and down in line with your upper body. Repeat 8 times on each side.

Back of thigh toners

4 Lie flat on the floor with your head resting on your hands. Slowly bend one knee and lift one foot up behind you as far as it will go; try to touch your bottom. Lower it to the floor and repeat 4 times each side. Control both the up and down movement.

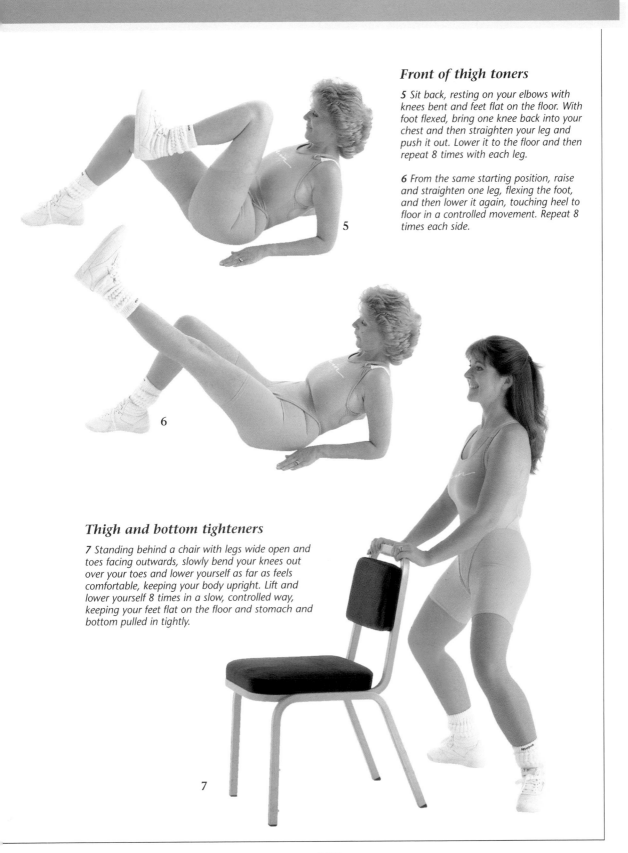

Front of thigh toners

5 Sit back, resting on your elbows with knees bent and feet flat on the floor. With foot flexed, bring one knee back into your chest and then straighten your leg and push it out. Lower it to the floor and then repeat 8 times with each leg.

6 From the same starting position, raise and straighten one leg, flexing the foot, and then lower it again, touching heel to floor in a controlled movement. Repeat 8 times each side.

Thigh and bottom tighteners

7 Standing behind a chair with legs wide open and toes facing outwards, slowly bend your knees out over your toes and lower yourself as far as feels comfortable, keeping your body upright. Lift and lower yourself 8 times in a slow, controlled way, keeping your feet flat on the floor and stomach and bottom pulled in tightly.

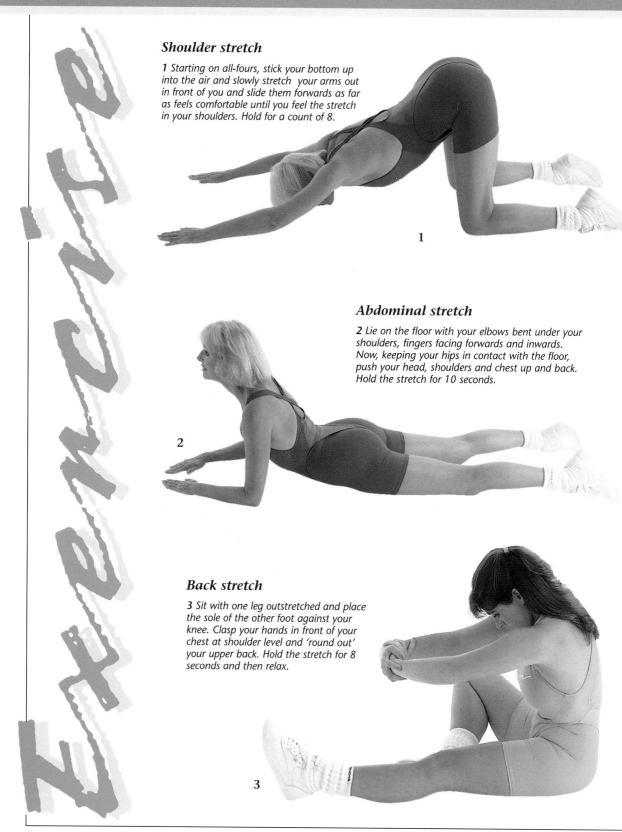

Shoulder stretch

1 Starting on all-fours, stick your bottom up into the air and slowly stretch your arms out in front of you and slide them forwards as far as feels comfortable until you feel the stretch in your shoulders. Hold for a count of 8.

Abdominal stretch

2 Lie on the floor with your elbows bent under your shoulders, fingers facing forwards and inwards. Now, keeping your hips in contact with the floor, push your head, shoulders and chest up and back. Hold the stretch for 10 seconds.

Back stretch

3 Sit with one leg outstretched and place the sole of the other foot against your knee. Clasp your hands in front of your chest at shoulder level and 'round out' your upper back. Hold the stretch for 8 seconds and then relax.

Bottom stretch

4 Sit up straight with your legs outstretched, and bend one knee and lift your foot over your other leg so that the foot is flat on the floor beside your bent knee. Place your opposite arm on the bent knee with your hand resting on the thigh. Support yourself with your other hand. Inhale and sit up straight, and then exhale and twist your upper body from the waist until you can look over your shoulder. Hold the stretch for 10 seconds and then repeat on the other side.

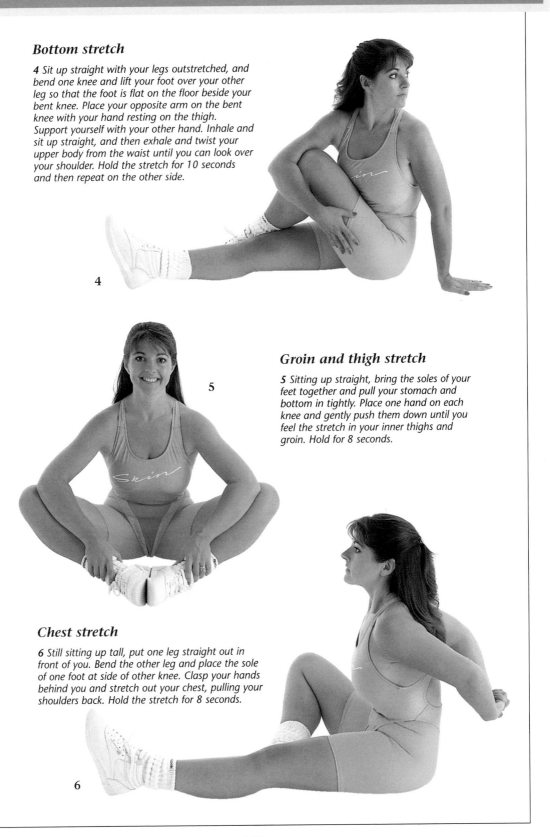

4

5

Groin and thigh stretch

5 Sitting up straight, bring the soles of your feet together and pull your stomach and bottom in tightly. Place one hand on each knee and gently push them down until you feel the stretch in your inner thighs and groin. Hold for 8 seconds.

Chest stretch

6 Still sitting up tall, put one leg straight out in front of you. Bend the other leg and place the sole of one foot at side of other knee. Clasp your hands behind you and stretch out your chest, pulling your shoulders back. Hold the stretch for 8 seconds.

6

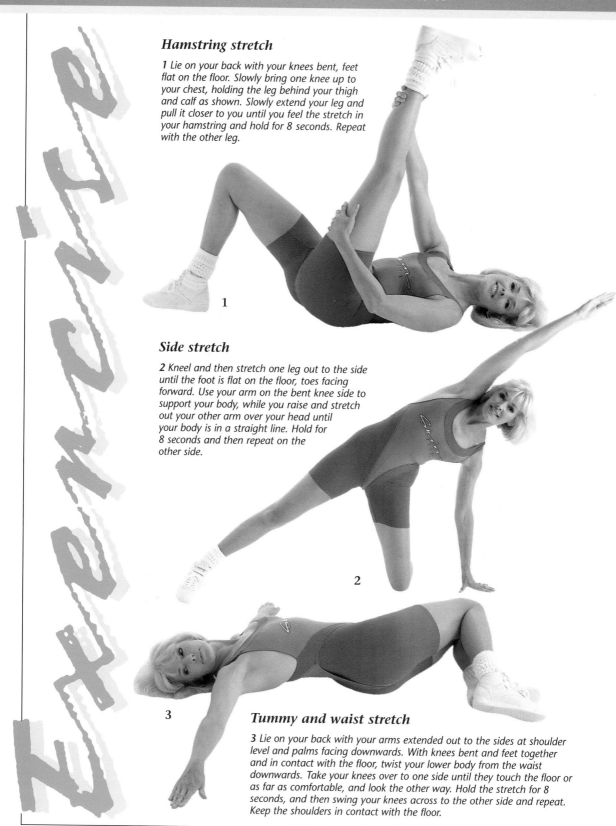

Hamstring stretch

1 Lie on your back with your knees bent, feet flat on the floor. Slowly bring one knee up to your chest, holding the leg behind your thigh and calf as shown. Slowly extend your leg and pull it closer to you until you feel the stretch in your hamstring and hold for 8 seconds. Repeat with the other leg.

Side stretch

2 Kneel and then stretch one leg out to the side until the foot is flat on the floor, toes facing forward. Use your arm on the bent knee side to support your body, while you raise and stretch out your other arm over your head until your body is in a straight line. Hold for 8 seconds and then repeat on the other side.

Tummy and waist stretch

3 Lie on your back with your arms extended out to the sides at shoulder level and palms facing downwards. With knees bent and feet together and in contact with the floor, twist your lower body from the waist downwards. Take your knees over to one side until they touch the floor or as far as comfortable, and look the other way. Hold the stretch for 8 seconds, and then swing your knees across to the other side and repeat. Keep the shoulders in contact with the floor.

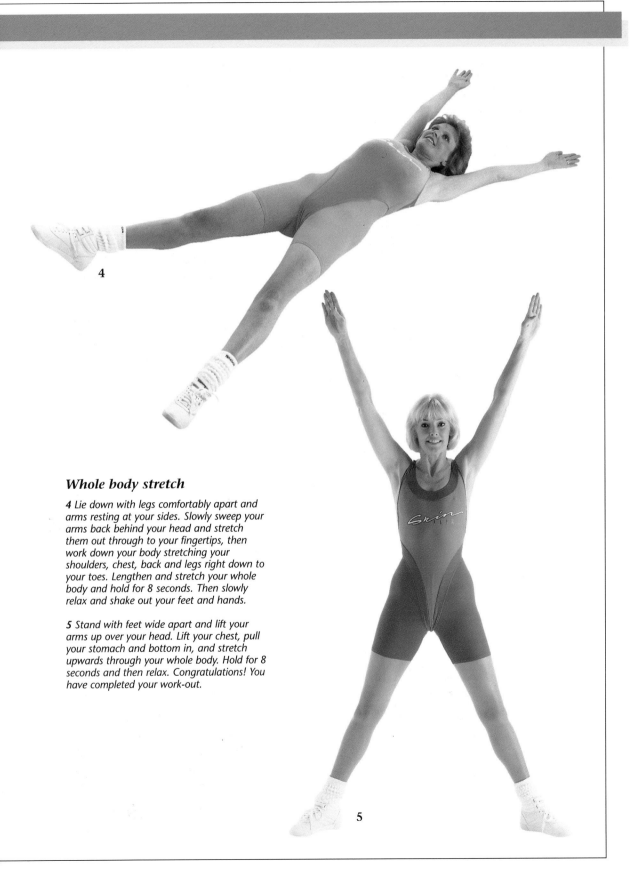

Whole body stretch

4 Lie down with legs comfortably apart and arms resting at your sides. Slowly sweep your arms back behind your head and stretch them out through to your fingertips, then work down your body stretching your shoulders, chest, back and legs right down to your toes. Lengthen and stretch your whole body and hold for 8 seconds. Then slowly relax and shake out your feet and hands.

5 Stand with feet wide apart and lift your arms up over your head. Lift your chest, pull your stomach and bottom in, and stretch upwards through your whole body. Hold for 8 seconds and then relax. Congratulations! You have completed your work-out.

OFF-THE-SHELF FOODS

You can stock up your store-cupboard with many healthy and low-calorie foods, e.g. canned beans and vegetables, rice and pasta. However, there are many convenience foods that are high in calories and you should choose a low-calorie alternative if possible, e.g. sardines in brine.

300g (10oz) canned cream of tomato soup
170 calories

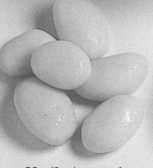

30g (1oz) mango chutney
80 calories

85g (3oz) boiled pasta (cooked weight)
100 calories

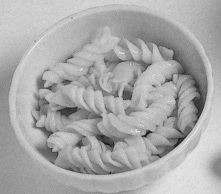

85g (3oz) canned new potatoes
54 calories

30g (1oz) canned sweetcorn kernels
35 calories

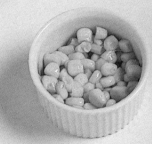

3 sweet dill pickles
6 calories

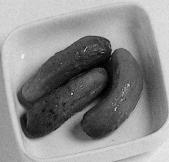

1 small can sardines in oil
300 calories

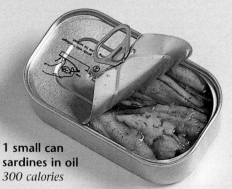

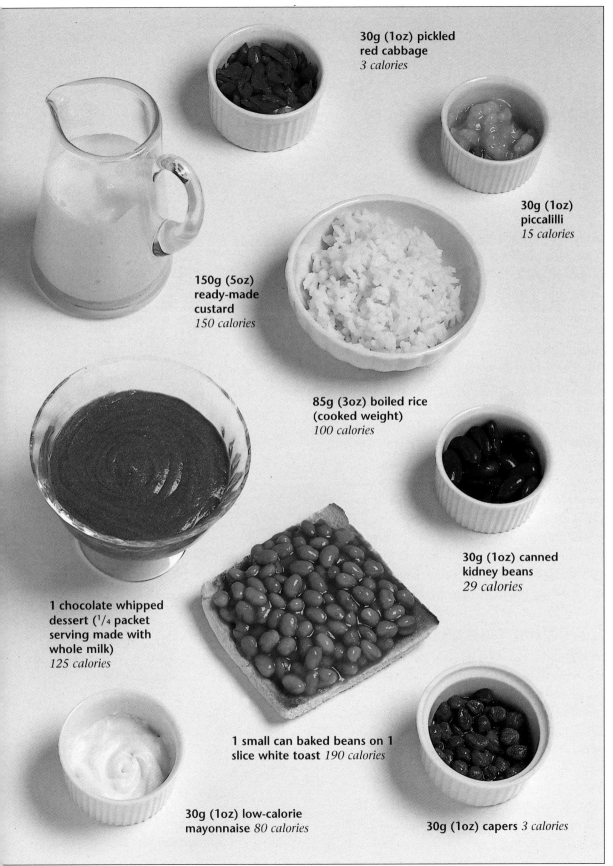

30g (1oz) pickled red cabbage
3 calories

30g (1oz) piccalilli
15 calories

150g (5oz) ready-made custard
150 calories

85g (3oz) boiled rice (cooked weight)
100 calories

30g (1oz) canned kidney beans
29 calories

1 chocolate whipped dessert (¹/₄ packet serving made with whole milk)
125 calories

1 small can baked beans on 1 slice white toast *190 calories*

30g (1oz) low-calorie mayonnaise *80 calories*

30g (1oz) capers *3 calories*

MAINTAINING YOUR IDEAL WEIGHT

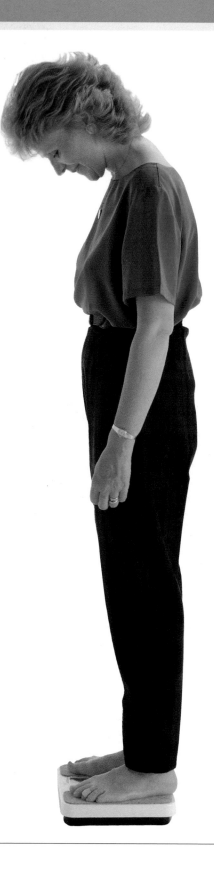

Congratulations if you have lost weight and have now reached your goal. You can feel proud of your new figure and all the hard work that went into achieving it. In this section of the book, we aim to show you how you can maintain your new weight and body shape for life.

The secret of weight maintenance is to avoid slipping back into your old eating habits; if this happens, then the overweight person lurking inside you will re-emerge and before you know it you'll be back where you started with all those miserable feelings.

It's now time for you to move out of dieting mode and into weight maintenance mode. Your aim during the next few weeks is not to measure your success in terms of weight loss on the scales, but in terms of increasing your daily calorie intake while still keeping those pounds at bay.

Increasing your calories without gaining weight

If you have tried to diet in the past, you will know only too well that you have to prepare yourself mentally for the challenge. With weight maintenance, the same rules apply. For perhaps the first time in your life, you will now have to learn to eat 'normally' without being driven to food for a whole host of reasons other than hunger. During maintenance, it is inevitable that you will be wary of eating foods that you could not control before, but your aim now is to remember that you really can eat anything, albeit in moderation.

In time, you will become less anxious about accounting for every calorie that passes your lips. Instead, you will be able to control your feelings and your food intake so that it will no longer be the all-consuming battle with which you have struggled in the past. It is a well-known fact that losing weight is simple – it's keeping those pounds at bay that is the true measure of a successful dieter!

While following our diet, you have learnt about eating more healthy, slimming food, and you should continue eating this way during maintenance. To maintain her weight, an average woman, i.e. one who is about 5ft 4in tall, between 19 and 50 years old and trying to maintain a weight of between 9st 7lbs and 10st, should consume approximately 1950 calories per day.

However, few of us are average, and, depending on our age, height and level of activity, we may need to eat anything between 1,700 and 2,400 calories per day for a woman; between 2,000 and 3,000 for a man. Now in order to maintain your weight, you have to find out what is the right calorie intake for you.

You can do this by gradually increasing the calories you consume until you find the correct intake to maintain your new healthy weight on a long-term basis. You will find some basic guidelines to help you below.

Adjusting your calorie intake

There are two ways of doing this. One way is to gradually move up one level of calories at a time each week until you reach the 1,650 calorie level in this book. If you find

Maintenance Guidelines

■ Don't snack or eat 'on the hoof'. Continue sitting down to proper meals and eating your food slowly. Savour every mouthful instead of bolting it down.

■ Keep fatty and sugary foods as occasional treats – not part of your normal daily food intake. Cakes, crisps, biscuits, sweets, pastries and chocolate are the foods that probably helped you to gain weight. You can still eat these, but in moderation.

■ Choose low-fat alternatives to full-fat foods whenever possible. So continue eating skimmed milk, low-fat cheeses, diet yogurts and low-fat spreads.

■ Don' t eat unless you are hungry, and don't waste calories on meals and food that you don't want. Left-overs may be better in the waste bin than in your stomach.

■ Try not to eat for comfort, e.g. when you are feeling upset, tired or under stress. Sort out the problem itself and do something positive about it. Overeating will only add to your problems – it will not make them disappear.

■ If a food is too tempting to stop at one portion, then don't start! Eat foods you can control.

■ Don't panic if you gain a couple of pounds. This is quite normal while your body is adjusting to your new maintenance mode; it is nothing to worry about. Nor does it mean that you will not be able to increase your level of calorie intake long-term.

■ Dress slim! Look slim! Treat yourself to some new clothes, a new hairstyle or a beauty make-over. Your pleasure and confidence in the 'new you' will help you to stay that way.

that you stabilize at one level or, indeed, slightly gain weight then you should continue on this level until your body adjusts and eventually allows you to lose weight again.

When you reach the 1,650 calorie intake and your weight stabilizes, you can then allow yourself an additional 1,000 calories a week to spend when and how you wish. It is at this point that the 'two off, five on' system may come into play. For example, you can choose to spend these extra bonus calories at the weekend. Of course, you don't have to do this, and you can spread them out across the week. Whatever your decision, your aim is the same: to increase your intake of calories without gaining weight.

You can continue increasing your weekly calorie intake by 1,000 calories until you reach a level that is right for maintaining your body weight. This process may take several weeks, depending upon how much weight you have lost. Careful weight maintenance will ensure that the building blocks are in place for the future, so don't try to rush this interim stage. It is important to take it slowly, one step at a time; your future success will depend on it.

The second way is for you to have 1,000 bonus calories each week for you to spend as and when you wish. This will allow you, for example, to enjoy that yearned-for Chinese meal or favourite treat which you have been avoiding while following the diet. How you spend these calories is for you to decide. You can divide them over seven days, enjoy them all at the weekend, or spend them over as many days as you please.

A word of warning: you should try when possible to spend these calories on a variety of healthy foods as well as on your favourite treats. For example, calories spent on extra fruit, potatoes or bread will be better for you than calories spent on foods that are high in fat. It is these foods that are the dieter's downfall and carry the added risk of usually being wickedly tempting – one portion, mouthful or nibble may not be enough!

If you continue to lose weight consuming these 1,000 bonus weekly calories, then you should add a further 1,000 calories the following week and continue until your weight stabilizes.

Two off, five on

Once your weight has stabilized, this is another way to keep those pounds at bay. Few of us actually eat the same number of calories every day, and there are usually a couple of days a week when we like to eat a

Maintenance tip

Although it is hard to adjust to the fact, you need to eat more food now, especially if you are a large weight loser who is frightened of becoming overweight again. It is vital that you increase your calorie intake when you have achieved a healthy weight for your height, for if you don't do this, your body will adapt to a low-calorie intake, and if you suddenly increase this to a sensible level in the future you could gain weight rapidly. This is why it is a good idea to spread the process of adjusting your calorie intake over several weeks until you discover what is the right calorie intake for you to maintain your weight. Plan your extra calories as carefully as you plan your food – don't be a compulsive eater.

little more than usual. For most of us, these two days are Saturdays and Sundays when we are feeling more relaxed and sociable and it is harder to control the food we eat, but of course they could be any two days of the week.

Weekends and social occasions can be a dieter's downfall, and even when you have achieved your ideal weight, they may continue to be a problem. So why are weekends difficult for you? Is it because you entertain and like to cook gourmet meals? Or do you eat out or order in high-calorie take-aways? Do you go shopping and succumb to the temptations of the bakery counter in your local supermarket? Or do you like to relax with a few drinks?

Whatever your reason for eating more at weekends, there is no need to feel guilty. It usually takes two or three days of careful eating to offset one day of over-eating, so if you 'go careful' from Monday to Friday, you can indulge yourself at weekends with two days of more relaxed eating by using your extra 1,000 bonus calories (see opposite).

You operate the system like this: just eat carefully during the week, sticking to low-fat, healthy foods along the guidelines on page 131 and then you can afford to eat higher-calorie foods at the weekend if you wish. You have earned this, and as long as you make up for it on Monday you won't gain weight. If weekends are your problem, then this is one way of tackling it. The 'two off, five on' way of eating has helped many successful slimmers to maintain their weight years after they stopped dieting.

Exercise to stay slim

If you have been exercising regularly since

Maintenance tip

Sometimes, people who have lost weight still feel 'fat'. Even when they look in the mirror at their new slim-line figure, they mistakenly see a fat person in the reflection. This is not an uncommon experience, as our minds may take a while to get accustomed to the new body image that we see. Our mental adjustment to being slimmer and staying that way may take some time, and is often understated. Believe in yourself and your new body image. You can feel proud of your body and the effort it took to achieve your new figure. Don't waste all that hard work; it is worth working hard at maintenance too.

you started your diet, you shouldn't give up now just because you have achieved your optimum weight. By increasing your exercise level you can burn off any extra calories that you may consume. Exercise helps burn up excess calories and speeds up your metabolic rate so that your body doesn't turn food into fat. It helps firm up problem areas and keeps you trim and fit and feeling good about yourself

If exercise is already a part of your life, then you probably enjoy it and will continue working-out regularly in whatever way you prefer. If not, and you lead a very sedentary lifestyle, change your habits now. Turn to page 112 to find out how to set about it safely and gradually. Exercise can bring you many benefits and much pleasure, and it is an important weapon against weight gain. In conjunction with your new, healthy way of eating, it can help you to maintain your new shape for life.

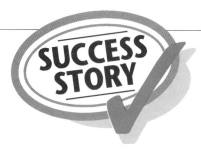

Donna Davies

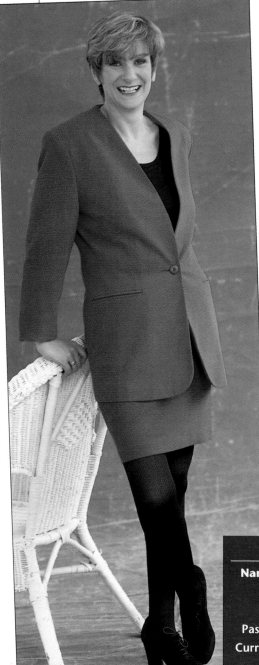

Donna Davies felt "old and tired all the time" before she joined her local Slimmer Clubs UK class and lost four stones. She used to wear baggy jumpers and leggings and didn't realise how big she was until she saw herself in some Christmas photographs.

Donna says: "I felt I owed it to myself to improve my overall appearance and health. Now that I have lost weight, I have far more energy and enjoy activities like gardening and walking. I have always been the life and soul of a party, but it's not a cover-up for my size any more. Now people are laughing with me, and not at me."

Donna was so delighted with her weight loss that she became a Slimmer Clubs Adviser. She has been successful at maintaining her weight and her new size 12 figure and wants "to encourage and motivate other people to enjoy their lives to the full as well. I get a lot of pleasure from seeing them achieve their goal too."

For the first time in her life, Donna feels that she has become a "complete person", and she is determined to stay that way.

FACT FILE

Name: Donna Davies
Age: 41
Height: 5ft 5in
Past weight: 13st 3lbs
Current weight: 9st 3lbs

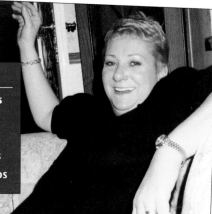

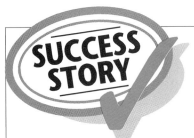

SUCCESS STORY

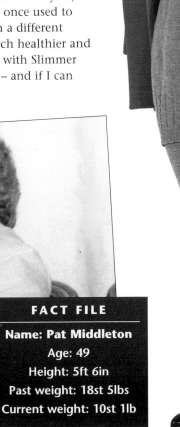

Pat Middleton

For more than 30 years Pat Middleton was known as 'fatty Patty', 'hippo' and 'barrel', but within 14 months of joining Slimmer Clubs UK, she had lost an amazing eight stones.

Pat says: "I tried everything from tablets and injections to hypnosis and acupuncture, but the truth is I never managed to educate myself about sensible eating until I joined Slimmer Clubs."

Thanks to her new healthier eating habits, Pat has maintained her weight for over a year, and it is hard to believe that she once used to squeeze into size 26 dresses! "I'm a different person. I love going out, I'm much healthier and more confident and I know that with Slimmer Clubs UK I will stay slim for life – and if I can stay slim, anyone can."

FACT FILE

Name: Pat Middleton
Age: 49
Height: 5ft 6in
Past weight: 18st 5lbs
Current weight: 10st 1lb

CALORIES IN EVERYDAY FOODS

BISCUITS

Sweet

per biscuit

Bourbon	70
Chocolate Chip Cookie, small	55
Chocolate Digestive, large	85
Chocolate Digestive, small	60
Custard Cream	65
Digestive, large	80
Digestive, small	50
Fig Roll	60
Fruit Shortcake	40
Garibaldi	40
Ginger Nut	40
Jaffa Cake	45
Kit Kat	110
Lemon Puff	75
Lincoln	40
Malted Milk	40
Marie	20
Morning Coffee	20
Nice	45
Penguin	127
Rich Tea	40
Rich Tea Finger	25
Shortbread Finger	100
Shortcake	65
Sponge Finger	25
Wafer, cream filled	30

Savoury

per biscuit

Cheese Sandwich, small round	45
Cheese Thin	20
Cornish Wafer	45
Cream Cracker	35
Matzo, large	75
Oatcake, small round	55
Rice Cake	30
Ryvita, Original or Dark Rye	25
Snack Cracker, small round	15
Water Biscuit, small	25
Water Biscuit, large	35

BREADS

per 30g (1oz)

Brown	65
Danish	68
French	80
Granary	70
Hovis	64
Lardy Cake	125
Malt	79
Rye	66
Soda	78
Softgrain	69
White	65
Wholemeal	64

per item

Bagel, large	225
Bagel, small	160
Bap, brown or white	140
Bap, wholemeal	135
Breadstick	20
Crisp Roll, per piece	40
Croissant, large	295
Croissant, small	175
Crumpet	75
Crusty Roll	130
Dinner Roll with Seeds	125
Finger Roll	100
Morning Roll	120
Muffin	150
Pikelet	50
Pitta Bread, white or wholemeal, large	180
Pitta Bread, white or wholemeal, small	90
Scotch Pancake	80
Soft Roll	130
Teacake	150

BREAKFAST CEREALS

per 30g (1oz) or as stated

Bran Flakes	90
Corn Flakes	110
Fruit & Fibre	110
Muesli	115
Porridge Oats, dry weight	115
Puffed Rice	105
Puffed Wheat	100
Shredded Wheat, each	78
Weetabix, each	65

CAKES

per 30g (1oz)

Angel Layer	120
Bakewell Tart	120
Battenburg	115
Cherry Genoa	105
Chocolate covered Swiss Roll	120
Dundee	105
Fruit	100
Ginger	115
Madeira	115
Sultana	105
Swiss Roll with jam	105
Swiss Roll with jam and buttercream	110
Victoria Sponge, with cream and jam	140
Walnut Layer	120
Wedding/Xmas Cake	105

per item

Almond Slice	150

Apple Pie, small	200
Bath Bun	170
Cherry Bakewell	200
Chocolate covered Mini Roll with buttercream	120
Chocolate covered Mini Roll with jam	115
Cup Cake	150
Current Bun, small	150
Custard Tart, small	200
Danish Pastry	350
Doughnut, jam filled	250
Doughnut, fresh cream	350
Eccles Cake	275
Flapjack Finger	175
Fondant Fancy	100
Hot Cross Bun	190
Jam Tart	125
Junior Jam Roll	100
Meringue Nest	60
Mince Pie, small	200
Rock Cake	200
Scone, with fruit	175
Trifle Sponge	80

CEREALS

General products

Flour, per 30g (1oz)

Chapati	98
Cornflour	104
Soya, fat reduced	103
Soya, full fat	131
Wheatmeal	95
White	103
Wholemeal	93

Pasta

per 30g (1oz)
(Dry weight, or as stated)

Chinese Egg Noodles	96
Egg Pasta	113
Egg Pasta, boiled	40
White or Coloured, boiled	40
Wholemeal	98
Wholemeal, boiled	35

Pastry

per 30g (1oz)

Choux, baked	97
Filo, as sold	80
Flakey, baked	165
Flakey, raw	128
Puff, frozen, raw	114
Shortcrust, baked	155
Shortcrust, raw	135
Wholemeal Shortcrust, baked	145
Wholemeal Shortcrust, raw	125

CRISPS AND SNACKS

per 30g (1oz), or as stated

Bombay Mix	150
Crisps	160
Crisps, per 25g bag	135
Crisps, lower fat	145
Crisps, lower fat, per 25g bag	120
Peanuts	175
Peanuts and Raisins	140
Popcorn, Butterkist	110
Popcorn, Toffee	120
Sesame Seeds	180
Sunflower Seeds	175
Tortilla Chips	130
Trail Mix	125
Twiglets, each	4

Rice and Grains

per 30g (1oz)
(Dry weight, or as stated)

Barley	103
Basmati Rice	105
Brown Rice	106
Brown Rice, boiled	43
Bulghur (Cracked Wheat)	103
Couscous	101
Millet	96
Sago	104
Semolina	103
Tapioca	106
Wheat Bran	60
Wheat Germ	107
White Rice	103
White Rice, boiled	38
Wild Rice	104

DAIRY

Cheese

per 30g (1oz), or as stated

Austrian or Bavarian Smoked	90
Babybel	94
Boursin	122
Brie	95
Caerphilly	110
Camembert	89
Cheddar	120
Cheddar, half fat	80
Cheese Spread	80
Cheese Triangles, half fat	30
Cheshire	110
Cottage Cheese	25
Cream Cheese	130
Curd Cheese	50
Danish Blue	105
Derby	118
Dolcelatte	110
Double Gloucester	118
Edam	95
Emmental	115
Feta, medium fat	70
Gorgonzola	105
Gouda	110
Gruyère	120
Lancashire	110
Leicester	118
Mascarpone	135
Mozzarella	85
Parmesan	135
Port Salut	98
Processed Cheese Slices, each	63
Processed Cheese Slices, half fat, each	40
Quark	45
Quark, skimmed milk	20
Roquefort	109
Roule	90
Soft Cheese, half fat	50
Stilton	120
Wensleydale	111

Cream

per 30g (1oz)

Aerosol	90
Clotted	170

Crème Fraîche	115
Double	130
Half	45
Single	60
Soured	62
Sterilized, cream	70
Whipping	110

Milk

Dried skimmed milk powder, per 30g (1oz)	100
Evaporated Milk, unsweetened, per 15ml tbsp	23
Semi-skimmed, per 30ml (1fl oz)	13
Semi-skimmed, per pint	260
Semi-skimmed, per 500ml carton	245
Skimmed, per 30ml (1fl oz)	10
Skimmed, per pint	195
Skimmed, per 500ml carton	175
Unsweetened Soya Milk, per 500ml carton	200
Whole, per 30ml (1fl oz)	20
Whole, per pint	380
Whole, per 500ml carton	340

Yogurt & Fromage Frais

Fromage Frais, 8% fat, per 15ml tbsp	18
Fromage Frais, 8% fat, per 30g (1oz)	35
Fromage Frais, 8% fat, flavoured per 100g carton	135
Fromage Frais, fat free, per 15ml tbsp	7
Fromage Frais, fat free, per 30g (1oz)	14
Fromage Frais, fat free/ diet, flavoured per 100g carton	50
Yogurt, low fat, natural per 30g (1oz)	17
Yogurt, low fat, natural per 15ml tbsp	8
Yogurt, very low fat/diet, flavoured per 125g carton	60

Yogurt, Greek, per 30g (1oz)	35

DESSERTS

Average calories

Black Forest Gateau, frozen, per 30g (1oz)	135
Custard, made with skimmed milk, per 150ml (1/4 pint) serving	100
Custard Powder, per 30g (1oz)	105
Fruit Pies, per 30g (1oz)	75
Ice cream, per 30g (1oz)	55
Ice cream, reduced calorie, per 30g (1oz)	40
Instant Dessert, Made with skimmed milk, per 85g (3oz) serving	90
Jelly, per 150g (5oz) made up	100
Jelly, sugar free, per 150g (5oz) made up	10
Lemon Meringue Pie, per 30g (1oz)	95
Sorbet, per 30g (1oz)	35
Sponge Puddings, per 30g (1oz)	100
Treacle Tart, per 30g (1oz)	110

DRINKS

Beverages

Cocoa Powder, per 30g (1oz)	95
Coffee	neg
Drinking Chocolate Powder, per 30g (1oz)	110
Tea	0
Tea, Fruit or Herbal, per cup	2
Water	0

Carbonated Drinks

per 330ml can

Cola	130
Cola, Diet	1
Cream Soda	80
Ginger Beer	100

Lemonade	80
Lemonade, Diet	1
Orangeade	100
Orangeade, Diet	3

Juices

per 100ml (3½ fl.oz)

Apple	45
Grape	65
Grapefruit	30
Orange	40
Pineapple	45
Tomato	25

Mixers

per 100ml (3½fl.oz)

American Ginger Ale	40
American Ginger Ale, diet	1
Bitter Lemon	35
Bitter Lemon, diet	2
Dry Ginger	20
Dry Ginger, diet	1
Soda Water	0
Tonic Water	25
Tonic Water, diet	1

Drinks, alcoholic

Aperitifs, per 50ml pub measure

Vermouth, Bianco	80
Vermouth, Dry	60
Vermouth, Extra Dry	55
Vermouth, Rose	75
Vermouth, Rosso	80

Beer

per 275ml (½ pint)

Bitter or Pale	90
Brown Ale	90
Mild	70
Stout	105
Strong Ale	205
Low Alcohol	60

Cider

per 275ml (½ pint)

Dry	100
Sweet	120
Vintage	285

Lager

per 275ml (½ pint)

Extra Strong	200
Normal Strength	85
Low Alcohol	50

Liqueurs

per 25ml pub measure

Advocaat	70
Cherry Brandy	65
Cointreau	80
Cream Liqueurs	85
Crème de Menthe	80
Grand Marnier	80
Kirsch	50
Tia Maria	75

Madeira, Port, & Sherry

per 50ml pub measure

Madeira	75
Port, Ruby or Tawny	75
Port, Vintage	85
Sherry, Dry	60
Sherry, Extra Dry	50
Sherry, Medium	65
Sherry, Sweet or Cream	75

Spirits

per 25ml pub measure

Brandy, Gin, Rum, Vodka or Whisky	50

Wine

per 150ml (5fl oz)

Champagne	105
Ginger	200
Low Alcohol	40
Red	95
Rose	100
White, dry	90
White, medium	105
White, sparkling	105
White, sweet	130

EGGS

Size 1	95
Size 2	90
Size 3	80
Size 3, white only	15
Size 3, yolk only	65
Size 4	75
Size 5	70

FATS

per 30g (1oz) or as stated

Butter	225
Ghee	270
Lard	270
Low-fat Spread	120
Margarine	225
Oil, all types	270
Oil, per 15ml tbsp	135
Suet, shredded	250
Sunflower Margarine	225
Very Low-fat Spread	80

FISH

per 30g (1oz) or as stated

Anchovies, per drained fillet	10
Bass	35
Bloaters, filleted	72
Caviar	73
Caviar, lumpfish	30
Cockles, shelled	14
Cod's Roe	25
Cod, fillet, raw	23
Cod, fillet, steamed	25
Coley, (Saithe), raw	22
Coley (Saithe), steamed	28
Crabmeat	37
Eel	48
Fish Finger, each, grilled	50
Haddock, fillet, raw	22
Haddock, fillet, steamed	29
Hake	24
Halibut, fillet, raw	27
Halibut, fillet, steamed	38
Herring, fillet, grilled	59
Herring, fillet, raw	69
Hoki	25
Kipper, fillet, baked or grilled	60
Kipper, on bone, baked or grilled	33
Lobster, meat only	35
Mackerel, fillet, fried or grilled	56
Mackerel, fillet, raw	66
Mackerel, on bone, fried or grilled	40
Monkfish	20
Mullet	37
Mussels, in shell	9
Octopus	22
Oysters, shelled	16
Pilchards in Tomato Sauce	37
Plaice, fillet, raw or steamed	28
Prawns, in shell	13
Prawns, peeled	32
Rock Salmon (Huss)	37
Rollmops	59
Salmon, pink, canned	40
Salmon, red, canned	50
Salmon, smoked	49
Salmon, steaks, raw	54
Salmon, steaks, steamed	58
Sardines in Tomato Sauce	53
Sardines, fresh	52
Scallops, steamed	31
Scampi, fried in breadcrumbs	94
Skate	30
Sole, fillet, raw	24
Sole, fillet, steamed	27
Squid	24
Trout, fillet or smoked fillet	40
Trout, on bone	26
Tune in Brine, canned, drained	29
Tuna in Oil, canned, drained	55
Whelks, in shell	4
Whelks, shelled	27
Whitebait, fried	160
Whiting, filled, steamed	27
Winkles, in shell	4
Winkles, shelled	21

FRUIT

per 30g (1oz) weighed with skin, stones, pips, or as stated

Apple, cooking	7
Apple, eating	12
Apricot	8
Apricots, dried	52
Avocado	39

Banana	18
Banana, flesh only	27
Blackberries	7
Blackcurrants	8
Cherries	11
Clementines	8
Cranberries	4
Currants, dried	76
Damsons	10
Dates, dried	65
Dates, fresh, per date	15
Figs, dried	65
Figs, fresh	12
Gooseberries, cooking	5
Gooseberries, dessert	10
Grapefruit	6
Grapes	16
Greengages	13
Guava, canned in syrup	17
Guava, fresh	7
Kiwi	12
Kumquats	20
Lemon	4
Lime	10
Loganberries	5
Lychees, each	8
Mango	16
Melon, Cantaloupe or Charentais	4
Melon, Galia or Ogen	5
Melon, Honeydew or Yellow	5
Melon, Watermelon	3
Mixed Peel, dried	66
Nectarine	10
Olives, small, each	3
Olives, large, each	5
Orange	7
Passion Fruit	6
Papaya	8
Peach	9
Pear	10
Pineapple, flesh only	12
Plantains, flesh only	32
Plums	10
Pomegranate	10
Prunes, dried with stones	37
Prunes, dried without stones	46
Quince	7
Raisins	78

Raspberries	7
Rhubarb	2
Satsuma	7
Sharon Fruit	20
Star Fruit	10
Sultanas	71
Tangerine	7

MEAT

per item

Bacon, back rasher, trimmed, grilled	40
Bacon, streaky rasher, grilled	50
Bacon Chop, trimmed, grilled	140
Bacon or Gammon Steak 100g (3½oz), trimmed, grilled	105
Beefburger, grilled	115
Beefburger, low fat, grilled	80
Beefburger, Quarter-pounder, grilled	240
Chicken Drumstick, grilled, skin on	75
Chicken Drumstick, grilled, skin off	60
Chicken Quarters, 250g (9oz) raw weight, roasted, skin on	360
Chicken Quarters, 250g (9oz) raw weight, roasted, skin off	190
Chicken Thigh, grilled, skin on	160
Chicken Thigh, grilled, skin off	90
Duck Breast, no fat or skin	160
Lamb Chop, 115g (4oz), raw weight, grilled	200
Pork Loin Chop, 115g (4oz), trimmed of fat, on bone, raw weight, grilled	190
Sausage, Pork, large, grilled	140
Sausage, Pork, small, grilled	75
Sausage, Pork, large,	

low fat, grilled	115
Sausage, Pork, small, low fat, grilled	55

Beef

per 30g (1oz)

Braising Steak, raw	50
Braising Steak, raw, extra lean	43
Brisket, boiled, lean and fat	92
Fillet Steak, weighed raw, grilled	42
Mince, raw	62
Mince, weighed raw, fried and drained	48
Mince, fried and drained	75
Mince, extra lean, raw	49
Mince, extra lean, weighed raw fried and drained	42
Mince, extra lean, fried and drained	55
Minute Steak, raw	38
Rib, lean and fat, roast	100
Rump Steak, lean only, weighed, raw, grilled	44
Silverside, roast, lean only	50
Sirloin Steak, weighed raw, grilled	57
Stewing Steak, raw	50
Topside, roast, lean only	50

Chicken

per 30g (1oz)

Breast meat, raw	33
Breast meat, poached	46
Breast meat, roast	41
Leg meat, raw	36
Leg meat, poached	58
Leg meat, roast	44

Delicatessen Meats

per 30g (1oz)

Bierwurst	92
Black Pudding, fried	89
Brawn	46
Chopped Ham & Pork	83
Corned Beef	68

Frankfurters	80
Garlic Sausage	83
Ham Sausage	45
Ham, Boiled, lean only	50
Ham, canned or vac-pack, lean only	30
Ham, Shoulder, canned or vac-pack	35
Haslet	73
Liver Sausage	91
Luncheon Meat	89
Mortadella	83
Parma Ham, lean only	53
Pastrami, lean only	62
Polony	83
Pork Boiling Ring	142
Pork Loin	40
Salami	130
Saveloy	77
Scotch Egg, each	300
Turkey Breast	30
Tongue	87

Game

per 30g (1oz)

Grouse, meat only, roast	35
Rabbit, meat only, raw	35
Rabbit, meat only, stewed	53
Rabbit, weighed on bone, stewed	27
Venison, roast	57

Lamb

per 30g (1oz)

Breast, roast	125
Leg, raw, lean only	39
Leg, roast, lean only	58
Mince, raw	63
Mince, weighed raw, fried and drained	48
Shoulder, roast, lean and fat	90
Shoulder, roast, lean only	58

Offal

per 30g (1oz)

Heart, lamb	34
Heart, ox	32
Heart, pig	29
Kidney	26

Liver, calf	46
Liver, chicken	39
Liver, lamb	53
Liver, ox	50
Liver, pig	46
Oxtail, weighed on bone, stewed	26
Sweetbreads	39
Tongue, lamb	57
Tripe	30

Pork

per 30g (1oz)

Belly or Streaky, weighed, raw grilled	125
Escalopes, fully trimmed, raw	33
Fillet or Tenderloin, raw	33
Leg, raw, lean only	36
Leg, roast, lean only	55
Mince	57
Mince, weighed raw, fried and drained	52
Shoulder, roast, lean and fat	95
Shoulder, roast, lean only	52

Turkey

per 30g (1oz)

Breast meat, raw	30
Breast meat, roast	38
Leg meat, raw	33
Leg meat, roast	42

Veal

per 30g (1oz)

Fillet or Escalope, raw	31

NUTS

shelled per 30g (1oz)

Almonds	185
Brazil	205
Cashew	185
Chestnuts	51
Coconut, creamed block	200
Coconut, desiccated	180
Hazelnuts	195
Macadamia	225
Peanuts	175
Pecans	210

Pine Nuts	210
Pistachios	190
Walnuts	205

STORE CUPBOARD

Miscellaneous per 30g (1oz), or as stated

Baker's Yeast, dried	50
Baker's Yeast, fresh	15
Beef Extract, per 5ml tsp	20
Curry Powder	70
Custard Powder	105
Cornflour	105
Gelatine Powder	102
Gravy Powder	80
Jelly Cubes	80
Soy Sauce, per 15ml tbsp	10
Stuffing Mix, dry weight	115
Sugar	115
Tomato Purée, per 15ml tbsp	10
Vinegar	1
Worcester Sauce, per 15ml tbsp	10
Yeast Extract, per 5ml tsp	20

Sauces, Pickles & Dressings

per 15ml tbsp, or as stated

Apple Sauce, sweetened	18
Apple Sauce, unsweetened	10
Brown Sauce	15
Cocktail Cherries, each	10
Cranberry Sauce	20
French Dressing	80
French Dressing, oil-free	5
Horseradish	15
Horseradish, creamed	25
Mango Chutney	40
Mayonnaise	110
Mayonnaise, reduced-calorie	40
Mint Jelly	35
Mint Sauce	3
Mixed Pickle, per 30g (1oz)	5
Mustard Powder, per 30g (1oz)	130
Mustard, English, per 5ml tsp	10
Mustard, French, per 5ml tsp	5

Piccalilli	12
Pickled Onions, per 30g (1oz)	5
Red Cabbage, per 30g (1oz)	6
Redcurrant Jelly	35
Salad Cream	50
Salad Cream, reduced-calorie	20
Tartare Sauce	40
Tomato Ketchup	15

Spreads

per 30g (1oz) or as stated

Chocolate Hazelnut Spread	170
Chocolate Spread	100
Golden Syrup	85
Honey, per 5ml tsp	20
Jam	85
Jam, low sugar	40
Lemon Curd	85
Marmalade	85
Molasses	86
Pâté, Ardennes	105
Pâté, Brussels	95
Peanut Butter	190
Tahini	180
Treacle	85

SWEETS AND CHOCOLATES

per 30g (1oz), or as stated

Boiled Sweets	110
Chewing Gum, per stick	10
Chewing Gum, sugar free, per stick	5
Chocolate, milk or plain	155
Fruit Pastilles	100
Fudge	120
Hard Gums	105
Honeycomb	85
Jellies	95
Liquorice	90
Liquorice Allsorts	105
Marshmallows	100
Mint Humbugs	120
Mints	115
Nougat	105
Rock	105
Sherbet Powder	100
Toffee	130
Wine Gums	100

VEGETABLES AND VEGETARIAN

per 30g (1oz)

Artichoke, Globe	5
Artichoke, Jerusalem	7
Asparagus	7
Aubergine	4
Beans, Baked in Tomato Sauce	22
Beans, Broad	23
Beans, Butter, boiled or canned	22
Beans, Green	7
Beans, Haricot, boiled	27
Beans, Kidney, boiled or canned	29
Beans, Runner	7
Beans, Soya, boiled	40
Beansprouts	9
Beetroot	13
Broccoli	9
Cabbage	7
Carrots	9
Cauliflower	10
Celery	2
Chickpeas, boiled or canned	35
Chicory	3
Chillies	6
Chinese Leaf	7
Corn on the Cob	19
Corn, Whole Baby Cobs	7
Courgettes	5
Cucumber	3
Eddoes	28
Endive	3
Fennel	3
Garlic	33

Garlic, per clove	2
Ginger, fresh	13
Horseradish	17
Kale	10
Kohlrabi	7
Leeks	6
Lentils, boiled	30
Lentils, dried	90
Lettuce	4
Mangetout	9
Marrow	3
Mooli	7
Mushrooms	4
Mustard & Cress	4
Okra	9
Onion	7
Onion, Spring, each	2
Parsley	10
Parsnips	18
Peas, frozen	20
Peas, Garden, canned	23
Peas, Mushy	23
Peas, Split, boiled	34
Peas, Split, dried	90
Peppers, Green	5
Peppers, Red, Yellow or Orange	10
Potatoes	21
Potatoes, chips, thick	55
Potatoes, chips, thin	80
Potatoes, New, canned	18
Potatoes, roast	43
Pumpkin	4
Radish	3
Shallots	14
Spinach	7
Spring Greens	9
Swede	7
Sweet Potato	24
Sweetcorn, canned	35
Textured Vegetable, Protein, dry weight	75
Tofu	25
Tomatoes	5
Turnips	7
Watercress	6
Yams	33

Slimmer Clubs UK Classes

At Slimmer Clubs UK we have been helping people to lose weight for 26 years. We understand only too well that dieting alone can sometimes be a struggle, and for that reason we provide in excess of 800 weekly weight loss classes nationwide. We know that dieting within a group is successful, and you too could discover that you can lose weight in our classes. The people who attend our classes find them informative, encouraging, motivational and, more importantly, fun!

If you go along to your local class, you will receive lots of help and support, and, with the help of other members and your Adviser, you will soon discover the way to diet sensibly and successfully.

Even when you have reached your ideal weight, we continue to offer you support and encouragement. We have a maintenance programme for you to follow, and as one of our privileged Gold Star Members, you will be able to attend your class once a month free of charge, provided that you stay within three pounds of your ideal weight.

If you would like details of your nearest class, call one of the following numbers today. You have nothing to lose but weight!

Slimmer Clubs UK Hotline:	0235 550700
Southern England:	0305 264314
Central England:	0235 550700
North-west England:	0942 518842
North-east England:	0325 381247
Scotland:	0325 381247

Or you can write to our Head Office at:

Slimmer Clubs UK
Cholswell Court
Cholswell Road
Abingdon
Oxon OX13 6HW

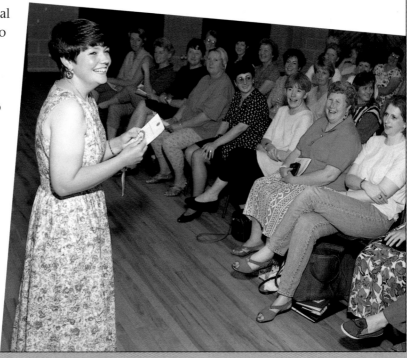

Recipe index